Developing Assessment Programs
for the
Multi-handicapped Child

Developing Assessment Programs
for the
Multi-handicapped Child

Edited by

JOSEPH N. MURRAY, Ph.D.

Coordinator
School Psychologist Training Program
Kent State University
Kent, Ohio

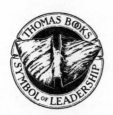

CHARLES C THOMAS • PUBLISHER
Springfield • Illinois • U.S.A.

Published and Distributed Throughout the World by
CHARLES C THOMAS ● PUBLISHER
Bannerstone House
301-327 East Lawrence Avenue, Springfield, Illinois, U.S.A.

© *1980, by* CHARLES C THOMAS ● PUBLISHER
ISBN 0-398-04052-4 (cloth)
ISBN 0-398-04076-1 (paper)
Library of Congress Catalog Card Number: 80-11756

Printed in the United States of America
V-R-1

Library of Congress Cataloging in Publication Data

Developing assessment programs for the multi-handicapped child.

Bibliography: p.
Includes index.
1. Handicapped children--Services for. 2. Handi-
capped children--Education. I. Murray, Joseph N.
[DNLM: 1. Handicapped. 2. Education, Special.
LC4015 D489]
HV888.D46   362.4'088054   80-11756
ISBN 0-398-04052-4
ISBN 0-398-04076-1 (pbk.)

To my mother and father for their ongoing guidance and support.

CONTRIBUTORS

Gerhardstein, Mark, M.Ed., Administrator, Deaf-Blind/ Multihandicapped Program, Ohio State School for the Blind, Columbus, Ohio

Knott, Gladys, Ph.D., Assistant Professor, Department of Special Education, Kent State University, Kent, Ohio

Murray, Elizabeth, M.Ed., School Psychologist Intern, Tallmadge City Schools, Tallmadge, Ohio

Murray, Joseph, Ph.D., Associate Professor, Coordinator, School Psychologist Training Program, Kent State University, Kent, Ohio

Robinson, Robert, Ph.D., Coordinator, Educational Assessment Project, Mid-Eastern Ohio Special Education Regional Resource Center, Akron, Ohio

Ross, Mike, Ed.D., Associate Professor, Department of Special Education, University of Akron, Akron, Ohio

PREFACE

LEGISLATION spawned in the seventies has mandated education for every school-aged child in the United States. Public Law 93-380 gave initial direction to a movement which guaranteed all children, regardless of the type, degree, or number of handicaps, a free education. Public Law 94-142 supported the philosophical intent of 93-380 by providing considerable financial support, but suddenly educators found themselves in a not-so-familiar position of having a legal mandate to meet with less than optimally trained persons to assume that responsibility. Many of the "unserved," school-aged population found, as a result of child search activities, a variety of moderate-to-severe handicaps which made them different from the child who had previously been served by traditional special education units. It became clear that many of these unserved children, along with those who were inappropriately served, must have educational programming provided which was specifically directed to their needs. With this realization having been established, educators began the tedious trial-and-error efforts required to put together meaningful special education programming that would allow for optimal education for the severe and/or multiply handicapped child.

As one might expect, a precursor of effective educational programming is accurate functional diagnostic assessment. In order for a child to receive appropriate instruction, training, and therapy, a functional assessment across all domains must be effected. Educators, being traditionally based, have been, and in many cases still are, oriented toward normative assessment — assessment that tends to describe children in statistical or numerical terms while paying little heed to children as functional human beings. It has been discovered over time that traditional normative assessment is relatively meaningless, and that a much more global approach to assessment is needed to comply with newly developed legislation and, most importantly, to help the severe and/or multiply impaired youngster.

This book has been developed out of five years of research on, and observation of, the evolution of programming for the severe and/or multiply handicapped child and will focus on assessment of this type of special youngster. It has been designed to be used by students training to work with the severe/multiply handicapped, as well as by those persons in the field who work with this population. Its intent is to provide the reader with information dealing with every facet of the assessment process as it relates to the severe and/or multiply handicapped population. In addition to dealing with numerous specific concepts and guidelines related to assessment of multihandicapped children, emphasis is placed on both normative and non-normative instrumentation which can be appropriately used with given handicaps. A description of traditional as well as newer instrumentation available for use with deaf or hearing impaired, language impaired, blind or visually impaired, physically handicapped, multiply handicapped, and handicapped children requiring vocational assessment is given in this book.

The book is the result of the cooperation and efforts of numerous persons. I especially wish to thank the contributing authors; all of whom are recognized as extremely knowledgeable people in the subject areas with which they have dealt.

J.N.M.

CONTENTS

Developing Assessment Programs
for the
Multi-handicapped Child

CHAPTER ONE

ASSESSING THE MULTI-HANDICAPPED CHILD: LEGAL MANDATES, ORGANIZATIONAL ISSUES, AND PROBLEMS

MARK GERHARDSTEIN, M.ED.

THE EVALUATION AND THE STUDENT: FIRST THINGS FIRST

CHILDREN identified as eligible for special education programs by virtue of their multi-handicapping conditions are no less children than other individuals. There is a critical need for professionals and parents to perceive students with handicaps as students (people) first. Too often, they are perceived in terms of their handicaps only and are plagued by a stereotypic and pitiful view of themselves. They are seen by others, and therefore see themselves, as a conglomeration of deficiencies. The perception of the multi-handicapped as people first is more difficult to hold and more important to keep in mind the severer the handicapping conditions of a student appear to be.

How does this relate to the assessment process? To a great degree, students with multi-handicaps become what we as parents, professionals, and as a society believe them capable of being. They become what we make available to them, both in physical and psychological resources. Therefore, before we begin to assess the strengths and weaknesses of those with multi-handicaps by looking at them from within their world, we should evaluate how we, as professionals, parents, and others may be creating the barriers to the realization of a stu-

The statements and opinions expressed herein do not represent the official views of the Ohio Department of Education or of the Ohio State School for the Blind.

dent's true potential from without. It is important in this time
of emphasis on compliance with the law, and during this time
of rapid improvement in the theory and technology available to
the educator, that two things be said first:

1. Evaluators must believe in multi-handicapped students as
   persons of much potential and dignity.
2. The evaluation process must be carried out in an environment as free from unduly restrictive professional or parental attitudes as possible.

ASSESSMENT AND THE LAW: (PUBLIC LAW 94-142)

"The Education for all Handicapped Children Act of 1975"
(Public Law 94-142) signed into law by President Gerald R.
Ford, November 29, 1975, has provided much legal direction for
the process of evaluating the child suspected of having handicaps. One result has been that between 1975 and the present
there have been a rash of state legislative and educational
policy changes intended to bring state and local government
agencies into compliance with this law and the ensuing federal
regulations governing the implementation of Part B of this act
as issued by the Department of Health, Education and Welfare
on August 23, 1977.

The Federal Regulations dealing with procedural safeguards,
Part B of the Education of the Handicapped Act, Title 45,
Subpart E, Sections 121a.500 to 121a.534, have much to say
about this evaluation process and should be read directly and
studied relative to their implications in the assessment process.
It is important to become directly familiar with the facts as
presented in the law and the regulations before venturing either
into interpretation or implementation. The purpose of this
section is to familiarize prospective evaluators with the requirements governing the evaluation process as they are set forth in
the law and the regulations, to extrapolate from these requirements what some of the implications for assessment of the
multi-handicapped are, and to suggest how some of the good
educational practices available for use in the assessment process
can be built into the evaluation procedures used.

Among the most significant aspects of the law related to

assessment is the requirement that all initial and reevaluation assessments of handicapped children shall be multi-factored. Section 121a.532 (d) and (f) states:

> (d) No single procedure is used as the sole criterion for determining an appropriate educational program for a child;
> (f) The child is assessed in all areas related to the suspected disability, including, where appropriate, health, vision, hearing, social and emotional status, general intelligence, academic performance, communicative status, and motor abilities.

Specifically related to the tests and other evaluation materials to be utilized in a Multi-Factored Evaluation (MFE), the Federal Regulations state, Section 121a.532 (a) (1) (2) (3); (b) (c):

> (a) Tests and other evaluation materials:
> (1) Are provided and administered in the child's native language or other mode of communication, unless it is clearly not feasible to do so;
> (2) Have been validated for the specific purpose for which they are used; and
> (3) Are administered by trained personnel in conformance with the instructions provided by their producer;
> (b) Tests and other evaluation materials include those tailored to assess specific areas of educational need and not merely those which are designed to provide a single general intelligence quotient;
> (c) Tests are selected and administered so as best to ensure that when a test is administered to a child with impaired sensory, manual, or speaking skills, the test results accurately reflect the child's aptitude or achievement level or whatever other factors the test purports to measure, rather than reflecting the child's impaired sensory, manual, or speaking skills (except where those skills are the factors which the test purports to measure);

Who must perform the MFE? Section 121a532 (e) states:

> (e) The evaluation is made by a multidisciplinary team or group of persons, including at least one teacher or other specialist with knowledge in the area of suspected disability.

Finally, how frequently is a multi-factored evaluation to take place? It must take place prior to the initial placement decision and as stated in Federal Regulations, Section 121a.534 (b):

(b) That an evaluation of the child, based on procedures
which meet the requirements under Section 121a.532, is conducted every three years or more frequently if conditions war-
rant or if the child's parent or teacher request an evaluation.

What are some of the implications of these regulations and
others related to the assessment process for the future and for
the behavior of those who would attempt to evaluate the multi-
handicapped?

1. The school psychologist has, in many states, born the sole
responsibility for the evaluation of students who were multi-
handicapped. These regulations require that more than one
person and more than one instrument be involved based on the
nature of the child's suspected disability. Achievement tests,
adaptive behavior measures, and criterion referenced and/or
developmental assessments conducted by teachers will often be
included as multi-factored evaluation data. Parents may be
asked to complete adaptive behavior measures, self-
administered behavior, and communication assessments and
will be asked to release any current medical and diagnostic
information available through such persons as neurologists,
pediatricians, or others. Additionally, reports from such persons as opthalmologists, audiologists, communications specialists, occupational and physical therapists, and others, as
needed, will be integrated into the information available prior
to the placement decision and will be available to the group of
persons involved in the writing of the initial Individualized
Education Program (IEP).

2. The process whereby a parent gives permission for a
multi-factored evaluation calls for parents to receive a written
and understandable copy of the rights they possess as outlined
in Federal Regulations, Section 121a.505.

The manner in which many school districts choose to make
initial contact with a family can be critical to the way the
parents perceive the process they are about to begin. The parents can be given the impression that they are about to engage
into an adversary relationship with the schools because of the
legal and formal nature of the material that is being given them
regarding their rights. They can also be presented their rights
in a manner which indicates that the information and the op-

tions presented are for their information and protection and are intended to give them greater options as a consumer of education. It is in emphasizing an enlightened consumer approach to the prior notice requirements of the law, particularly when these requirements are presented in oral or in written form, that the parents role in the educational evaluation process can be emphasized. The importance of parental input through participation at the IEP Conference cannot be emphasized enough.

It must be recognized that the parent can be a potentially valuable evaluation resource. Parents may provide essential and otherwise unavailable information. Their contribution to the process may also make the evaluation more multi-factored. The family will be more suitably prepared to implement certain aspects of the results of the evaluation process after having been involved in it as an essential member.

Additionally, the evaluation process, and specifically, the request for consent to evaluate are sure to bring out feelings in the parents to which the educator will need to respond. It is often helpful to ask several key questions before entering into the evaluation process with the parents of a multi-handicapped child:

   a. How and when did you first suspect your child had problems and may be handicapped in some way?
   b. What is the history of your relationship with the medical profession relative to your child's suspected problems? How does that history make you feel?
   c. What is the history of your relationship with other educators relative to your child's problems or suspected handicap? How does that history make you feel?
   d. What are some of the specific concerns that you would like this evaluation procedure to address? What are your hopes or feelings regarding this prospective evaluation?

Even the most legal and formal-sounding aspect of the law to the parents — the presentation of their rights — may be used as a mechanism to communicate a sense of respect for them as persons with rights, with feelings, and with valid observational skills. The professional should take much care to listen to the parents' needs and feelings, as well as to those of the child.

3. The requirement to test the specific areas of need related to each child's suspected disability is going to require more extensive assessments of the multi-handicapped student's persistent life needs. This will take place in order to determine the social, emotional, and academic performance of each student. The assessment of these Persistent Life Problem (PLP) areas will be conducted in the classroom using mostly criterion referenced resources. The continued emphasis on such areas of instruction as social problem solving, understanding the world of work, homemaking, and other independent living skills suggests that there be more criterion-referenced assessment done by teachers of the multi-handicapped. To this persistent life needs, assessment (appropriate norm-referenced academic assessments) can be added where appropriate.

4. The confidentiality of personally identifiable information is guaranteed in Sections 121a.560-576 of the Federal Regulations. A school district must have policies and procedures for the collection, disclosure, storage, and destruction of all personally identifiable educational records. There must be a list of those personnel who have free access to records and a procedure for others to follow in obtaining parental consent to view or obtain copies of these records. The parents may obtain copies of their child's educational records from the school district upon request, although, these copies may be provided on a fee basis. The parents or child, if the child is eighteen years old or older, may also request an educational agency to amend inaccurate or misleading records or records that violate the child's privacy or other rights. The educational agency must respond to requests for amendments to records within a reasonable period of time and, if in disagreement with the request, must inform the parents of their right to request a records hearing.

In addition to the regulations developed as a result of P.L. 94-142, the Family Rights and Privacy Act of 1974 and its accompanying regulations deals with issues related to educational records.

These confidentiality regulations have a direct bearing on the evaluation process. Parents must be informed of their rights as a part of the prior notice activities. The notice provided must be in written form and will include all of the parents' rights, including, but not limited to, those relating to the confidentiality of records. The parents will learn what will be written as a result of the evaluation, how they and others can gain access to these records, and what grievance procedures are available to them. In the course of the multi-handicapped student's career there are many significant evaluations conducted and reports filed. It is the intention of this section of the law to assure that educational records are accurate and are appropriately available to those parties involved in the educational process.

5. The requirement to provide a "free and appropriate public education" to all handicapped children contained in P.L. 94-142 has had a large impact on the school's role in providing diagnostic evaluation services; the school district may not be able to assure an appropriate placement based on the necessary multi-factored evaluation data. If there is a strong suspicion that any specialized area of functioning is deficient and contributes to a student's suspected educational handicap, then all the necessary diagnostic testing to identify the nature and educational implications of the suspected handicap should be conducted free of charge.

Many school districts are forming cooperative agreements with health department assessment projects, are working with their area university-affiliated facility, or are seeking out the financial and evaluation services of agencies such as the Bureau of Crippled Childrens Services when attempting to obtain a free and thorough multi-factored evaluation. In many cases, school districts have contracted with specific physicians for diagnostic services and refer parents to them for free assessments. If, in these instances, parents choose not to avail themselves of the free services being offered them, they may seek other evaluation resources at their own expense.

The evaluation resources necessary to identify the educational implications of a child's handicapping condition may bring forth data that suggests the need not only for special education but for one or more related services as well. Section 121a.13 (a) Related Services, states:

> (a) As used in this part, the term "related services" means transportation and such developmental, corrective, and other supportive services as are required to assist a handicapped

child to benefit from special education, and includes speech
pathology and audiology, psychological services, physical
and occupational therapy, recreation, early identification, and
assessment of disabilities in children, counseling services, and
medical services for diagnostic or evaluation purposes. The
term also includes school health services, social work services
in schools, and parent counseling and training.

6. The section of the Federal Regulations dealing with the
administration of tests in a child's native language suggest that
evaluators will have to look carefully at the modes of communication used and understood by the multi-handicapped child.
"Native language" should be taken to mean the verbal or nonverbal language normally used by the parent of the child or by
those in the environment from which the child comes. It may
be that the native language is English, but the form of that
language is the total communication combination of oral and
manual communication, or an adapted Bliss Symbolics System.
Serious attention should be given to assessing multi-
handicapped children without discriminating against them due
to a lack of familiarity with the adapted forms of communication they have been taught. For example, how many school
psychologists can sign well enough to conduct a cognitive assessment of a deaf child who signs? Additionally, how many of
those who could not sign would recognize the value of using an
interpreter, such as the child's teacher or parent. Such persons
would not only help the test situation to be nondiscriminatory,
but they might make the child feel more comfortable with the
evaluation and more available to, and interested in, optimum
performance.

The unique communication history and needs of each child
must be carefully taken into account and built into the evaluation format, procedures, and instruments utilized with each
multi-handicapped child. (see Section 121a.9 and 121a.532(1)).

7. Frequently, testers will have to use parts of one assessment
and part of another. Adaptations of the instructions provided
by the producer will have to be made to adapt test items to the
unique circumstances created by the multi-handicapped child.
Much informal evaluation, observational, and criterion-
referenced data may be collected to supplement any normative

testing, which may have been appropriately selected and administered.

When the adaptation of a test to meet the unique needs of a child threatens its statistical validity or threatens the reliability of the data collected due to necessary adaptations in the test instructions, What should be done? Assuming that the best available assessments have been selected, there may be nothing to do but to document the manner in which the tests have had to be altered, combined, and reinterpreted based on each unique testing situation. Parents should be given a description of each evaluation procedure to be used as part of the request for permission to evaluate, and at this time, the potential advantages and limitations of the proposed procedures should be explained. There will never be a day when all of the needs of multi-handicapped children will be well integrated into two, five, or even ten packaged assessment products. The unique needs and characteristics of some children will always force adaptations in the best of instruments. These adaptations are what separates the professional from the automaton. They will often make the difference between a quality child study, based on maximum child performance, and the perfunctory one.

8. The evaluation data should be used to determine the student's strengths and weaknesses. The identification of these strengths, as they are accumulated from the referring teacher, the parent, and other members of the evaluation team, should help those present at the IEP Conference to establish the extent to which the child can participate in the regular education program. To relegate a student, whose educational handicaps only effect part of his classroom schedule, to total segregation is violating his right to a placement in the least restrictive environment. Each placement should be based on a careful analysis of the student's assessed needs. The identification of a child as educationally handicapped should expand, not limit, the educational possibilities that are created.

9. The rules and regulations clearly require, in Section 121a.531, that all multi-factored evaluation procedures must be completed and all evaluation results made available to the group of persons making the placement decision before any

placement is made or IEP written. This has caused many large, cooperative, special education service centers to change their policy of enrolling children on less than complete evaluation data. Some children suspected of having multi-handicaps had previously been enrolled, as soon as the transportation from a nearby local school district could be arranged, and were evaluated after placement. Pre-placement evaluation has also forced the sending district to develop a greater understanding of what is being asked, since many of them are now much more involved in the evaluation process.

10. Based on each child's assessed needs, the special education program and all of the related services identified on the IEP must be provided. This is perhaps one of the most difficult issues for school districts. A child whose assessment data indicates the need for physical therapy two or three times a week should have that need reflected on the IEP. Many districts, however, do not have physical therapists, will not get reimbursed for money spent to purchase this service, and are without sufficient local funds to operate their existing programs much beyond what minimum standards require. The law is clear to indicate, however, that there is no valid reason, including a local lack of funds, which relieves the school district from providing those services identified as necessary during the course of the assessment and which are indicated on the IEP. (*see* Section 121a.301 (b)).

11. It is necessary to follow and document the activities related to each handicapped child, beginning with the referral indicating that a handicap is suspected, and including the evaluation, placement, annual review, and reevaluation activities. A documentation system is necessary to provide proof of appropriate implementation during the initial evaluation and placement and to assist in the systematic rescheduling and monitoring of annual reviews and reevaluations. There are many such child information management systems being developed to meet the needs of children and school personnel across the country.

The task of doing comprehensive initial and reevaluations on all identified handicapped students in keeping the required three-year cycle is forcing many school districts to develop a differential referral system for the use of school psychological services. In those instances where the purpose of a request for services does not involve the evaluation of a suspected handicap, but rather seeks such services as individual student counseling or applied behavioral analysis consultation, the prior notice evaluation and placement requirements of P.L. 94-142 do not apply. The development of a differentiated referral procedure can help referrals be processed and given precedence appropriately. Such a system will also encourage the continued delivery of a variety of school psychological services.

12. If a parent disagrees with an evaluation obtained by the public agency, the parent may indicate to the school district that they intend to seek an independent evaluation at the public's expense. If the public school district feels its existing evaluation is appropriate, they may initiate a hearing to determine the appropriateness of their evaluation. If a hearing officer finds their evaluation to be appropriate, the parents may obtain the requested additional evaluation data, but at their own expense. If the school district's evaluation is found to be inappropriate, the school district must provide an independent evaluation at no cost to the parent. Most agencies will seek a solution through mediation or by obtaining additional, free diagnostic evaluations from existing local, regional, or state resources. Where alternative, free diagnostic evaluation services may not be available to them, a school district will probably choose to pay for an independent evaluation if they feel that in so doing they could avoid incurring the large expense of a due process hearing.

13. It is the responsibility of the local school district, in conjunction with the state agency, to conduct intensive child find campaigns to identify, locate, and evaluate all handicapped children. This includes children from birth through age twenty-one who are either in or out of school (*see* Section 121a.220 and P.L. 93-380).

For the infant through two years of age and for the three or four-year-old handicapped child, in states where pre-school education of the handicapped child is not required by law, what should evaluation consist of? For these young children, a multi-factored evaluation would involve the same type of evaluation considerations that would be present for a school-age youngster. All areas of the suspected disability, which could contribute to the existence of an educational handicap, would need to be evaluated.

The school district may choose to make a special education placement for children three and four years of age if, according to all relevant federal and state laws, such an educational placement is not required.[1] If the evaluating local school district does not choose to make an educational placement, then they should provide, along with the explanation of the results of their evaluation, suitable mention of the existing early childhood education resources available locally that would be for the parents' consideration.

14. A group of persons making the placement decision should be knowledgeable about the child and the evaluation data that has been obtained. Section 121a.533 Placement Procedures states:

(a) In interpreting evaluation data and in making placement decisions, each public agency shall:

(1) Draw upon information from a variety of sources, including aptitude and achievement tests, teacher recommendations, physical condition, social or cultural background, and adaptive behavior;

(2) Insure that information obtained from all of these sources is documented and carefully considered;

(3) Insure that the placement decision is made by a group of persons, including persons knowledgeable about the child, the meaning of the evaluation data, and the placement options; and

(4) Insure that the placement decision is made in conformity with the least restrictive environment rules in Section 121a-550-121a-554.

(b) If a determination is made that a child is handicapped and needs special education and related services, an individualized education program must be developed

---

[1]For more details regarding the public school's responsibility for handicapped children from birth through four years of age see Title 45, Section 121a.300 of the Federal Rules and Regulations, Part B of the Education of the Handicapped Act.

for the child in accordance with Sections 121a.340-121a.349 of Subpart C.

Similarly, the law specifically requires that a direct link be established between the evaluation data that is obtained as part of the initial multi-factored evaluation and the writing of the initial IEP. The evaluation personnel, findings, and procedures, as they relate to the writing of an IEP for a child who has been evaluated for the first time, are dealt with in Section 121a.344 (b):

(b) *Evaluation Personnel.* For a handicapped child who has been evaluated for the first time, the public agency shall insure:

(1) That a member of the evaluation team participates in the meeting; or

(2) That the representative of the public agency, the child's teacher, or some other person is present at the meeting who is knowledgeable about the evaluation procedures used with the child and is familiar with the results of the evaluation.

There is clear indication that the IEP should follow directly from those areas wherein the student has been determined to be educationally handicapped. It is easy to see why the placement team meeting and the initial IEP meeting are often combined, because of the similarity in the required participants, their required knowledge of the child, and their ability to interpret the evaluation data. These combined meetings will usually involve a school psychologist, a teacher, the child's parent, a representative of the school district (other than the child's teacher) who is qualified to provide or supervise special education, and others, including the child, where appropriate.

15. Many school districts serve students from other districts in cooperative programs for multi-handicapped children. It appears clear in the law that the superintendent of the school district in which a student is a legal resident has the responsibility to make the placement of each handicapped child identified in the district. However, it is entirely possible that a school district may choose to delegate its responsibility to evaluate, to provide the annual review of the IEP, and to provide a three-year reevaluation to the school district in which the cooperative

program will take place.

In such instances, specific cooperative agreements should be established between the sending and the receiving district regarding the evaluation functions. Such questions as, who will assess and reassess; who will conduct annual reviews; who will retain and send copies of records relative to the evaluation and IEP process; and others should be spelled out in writing. Children placed in cooperative programs should always be followed in the child information management system of the school district of legal residence. The school district of the parent's legal residence, often called the local school district, is the key agency in this process. All requests for evaluation, requests for impartial due process hearings, or concerns about other matters of consequence to the continued desirability of the child's current IEP and placement are the responsibility of the local school district. Even if this district delegates its responsibility to evaluate to some other agency, they remain responsible for the continued appropriateness of the placement, the IEP, and for the appropriateness of the supporting evaluation data.

The issues raised by reference in this chapter to Public Law 94-142 can also be discussed as resulting from legal mandates in other legislation. The education of the handicapped amendments of 1974, Public Law 93-380, was the first major piece of federal legislation resulting from the increased awareness of the needs of handicapped children. This law requires the identification and evaluation of all children in the state suspected of being handicapped. It requires testing to be free of cultural bias, establishes the due process system, the right of the parent to obtain an independent evaluation, and a confidentiality policy requirement regarding educational records. Finally, this law includes the requirement for each state to adopt a state plan to contain the timetable regarding the provision of a full educational opportunity to each handicapped child. This plan was to also include specific procedures that were to be adopted to guarantee the provisions of the law.

The Vocational Rehabilitation Act of 1973, Section 504, states that no handicapped individual shall be denied participation in, or the benefits of, any programs or activities receiving federal assistance. Title 45, Section 84.35 of the Rules and Regulations governing the implementation of Section 504, deals specifically with all of the same requirements set forth in P.L. 94-142 regarding educational evaluation procedures to be used for suspected handicapped children. Additionally, many states have passed state laws to authorize the State Education Agency (SEA) to enforce the federal legislation and to create state plans governing the current and future direction of the state's special education programs.

What is it that all of these laws and regulations are trying to establish? They are trying to require people, to treat with creative dignity and respect, a population which has been, until the early 70s mostly overlooked and undereducated. In the evaluation process these laws provide support for a multi-faceted approach to discovering the needs of the multi-handicapped child. They require the respectful inclusion of the parent into the evaluation process as the consumer of education. They also provide parents with due process procedures if they feel that evaluation and/or placement procedures have been unmet, or the findings need to be changed. P.L. 94-142 is also trying to provide, at least partially, some of the financial resources it will require to implement the letter and the spirit of the mandates it contains.

Can positive educational attitudes result from legally required behavior? From the experience of persons entering the world of the multi-handicapped for the first time with an open mind, and with attitude of hopefulness, and with a healthy respect for the substantial lack of knowledge they are likely to possess, the answer is yes! Many positive attitudes have resulted from the required identification, evaluation, and placement of handicapped children across the country. However, there are educators who would place lesser value on the need for educating the multi-handicapped. An educator who believes that a multi-handicapped child deserves less than it would take for him/her to reach his/her full potential, or whose motivation for working with the multi-handicapped is not strong, should not be chosen to assume critical leadership positions. Not only are these attitudes contagious, but they are limiting. The law can do no more than to offer appropriate attitudes and behavior. Evaluation will always be a person-to-person process; a give and take; a willingness to go looking for each child individually with the purpose of communicating unconditional acceptance and finding the specific strengths and weaknesses upon which the future will depend. The purpose of the law, as it relates to evaluation and placement, is to add order, direction, and nondiscriminatory practices to parental and professional acceptance of each handicapped child.

DEFINITIONS OF MULTI-HANDICAPPED

The Federal Regulations governing the implementation of Part B of the Education of the Handicapped Act of 1975, contain a section which defines who it is that the law refers to as "Handicapped Children." Section 121a.5 (a) states:

(a) As used in this part, the term "handicapped children" means those children evaluated in accordance with Sections 121a.530-121a.534 as being mentally retarded, hard of hearing, deaf, speech impaired, visually handicapped, seriously emotionally disturbed, orthopedically impaired, other health impaired, deaf-blind, multi-handicapped, or as having specific learning disabilities, who because of those impairments need special education and related services.

Specifically related to the multi-handicapped, the regulations state in Section 121a.5 (b) (5):

(5) "Multi-handicapped" means concomitant impairments (such as mentally retarded-blind, mentally retarded-orthopedically impaired, etc.), the combination of which causes such severe educational problems that they cannot be accommodated in special education programs solely for one of the impairments. The term does not include deaf-blind children.

The purpose of the terms defined in this section of the regulations is to clarify who, for the purpose of the law, may be considered to be multi-handicapped.

Many states do not have state standards for special education, which indicate that students determined to be eligible as handicapped by virtue of their concomitant visual and auditory impairments are covered under separate standards from those relating to the rest of the multi-handicapped. In Ohio and Illinois, for example, the deaf-blind are covered under existing standards for the multi-handicapped. This is not to suggest that there should be no school age classes specifically for deaf-blind children. It means that for administrative purposes many states have, until this point, chosen to include the deaf-blind child under the same funding umbrella as other multi-handicapped children.

It is also true to say that there is variability in the placement of children whose educational handicaps are primarily resulting from the presence of "autisticlike" characteristics. The definitions section of the Federal Regulations includes the autistic child under the definition of those referred to as "seriously emotionally disturbed." In Ohio, the autistic child is served under the Standards for the Severe and/or Multiple Impairments. For the most part, these autistic children demonstrate learning problems, including autistic behaviors, social withdrawal, poor communication skills, and frequently concomitant mental retardation, that more appropriately place them in programs with the multi-handicapped. The decision to identify an autistic child as either seriously emotionally disturbed or multi-handicapped should not rest with the view taken regarding the etiology of a child's learning problems, but rather with the characteristics and educational needs unique to each child and common to those with whom he or she is placed.

It is clear that the multi-handicapped child should be identifiable as having some of the most severely educationally handicapping conditions. Children who are assessed as having two or more educational handicaps should not be placed in a multi-handicapped class unless it is clear that the programs serving children with either of their combined problems cannot meet their education needs. Many children with problems in vision, hearing, or with orthopedic disabilities also have disabilities in other areas. Some degree of mental retardation and some behavioral difficulties may also be present. The term "multi-handicapped," as it is associated with a child's disabilities, and as the identifier of a categorical educational program, is very restrictive. Program options for children with multi-handicaps should be available, not to protect, but to challenge each child enrolled to reach his or her full potential. Each child with multi-handicaps should, according to the law, be placed in the program for those with multi-handicaps in order for such a placement to be appropriate. Having two or more dis-abilities is not enough to make a person eligible, unless the placement team decides that the presence of concurrent educa-tional handicaps warrants the need for the special education program options available for those with multi-handicaps.

THE RELATIONSHIP BETWEEN ASSESSMENT AND THE ORGANIZATION OF THE INSTRUCTIONAL PROGRAM

The purpose of the educational program for the student with multi-handicaps should be to develop the attitudes, habits, and skills necessary to live and work during adult life. Many stu-dents will have to be taught how to initiate a variety of leisure time activities for themselves. All multi-handicapped students will have to learn to express their feelings and should be taught to think critically and to act as independently as possible.

Educational services should be available to the child with multi-handicaps and to the family of that child as early in the child's development as the identification and evaluation pro-cess can be undertaken. Parents will need support, encourage-ment, and direction in the appropriate developmental activities to undertake when a severely handicapped child is very young. Later, educators and parents, working as a team, will have to constantly evaluate whether they are underexpecting and thereby limiting the potential for growth. As the child gets older and it becomes evident that a strong academic orientation has either reached a point of diminishing returns or is not going to be appropriate, What should be done?

The initial placement evaluation and the later three-year reevaluations will focus on such domains as adaptive behavior related to communication, socialization, daily living skills, mo-bility, vocational training, and money use and management. There are the most critical areas of everyday functioning as members of a family, a community, a work environment, and as a member of society. The evaluation process has supposedly been thorough enough to evaluate all the areas related to the suspected disabilities. The real question then is whether the educational program resulting from this evaluation can free itself from the traditional role and set of circumstances associated with "being in school" enough to organize programming directed at the students' real needs.

The child with multi-handicaps may need to learn to dress and to eat independently; to manage and care for the domestic environment necessary to support adult living; and to access, to understand, and to negotiate the market place as well as the social options of the community. The classroom will suffice as the home base for the activities necessary to create a thorough instructional program, but will not be sufficient in itself. Moreover, the classroom will not have the flavor of an academic setting. There may be a learning center for food preparation, a mini-sheltered workshop, an area for instruction, or several current learning centers able to meet individual needs. The classroom space should be the teacher's architectural design of the assessment data and IEPs combined and should still have plenty of room for personal elaboration and creativity.

The room itself should provide structure and offer direction to the student in completing assignments and in making some independent choices about what to do next. It should provide space and opportunity to build on strengths as well as to provide work on disabilities. As many activities as possible of an expressive or social nature should be held in common with nonhandicapped peers. Examples of these include lunch, art, music, recess, movies, assemblies, and other nonacademic or academic instructional activities into which the students might analogously be placed.

Instruction will focus on real experiences as opposed to abstract concepts, and provision should be made for each objective to receive much practice before completion can be assured. Teaching from specifics to generalized principals or patterns of behavior requires careful planning and much variation in the persons, the settings, and the other general circumstances under which an objective might be experienced in real life.

There will be much more intensive, interdisciplinary and interagency involvement as well as a higher staff to student ratio than is characteristic of other special education programs. A teacher and two aides for six children would not be uncommon. Additionally, parents and other persons would frequently be encouraged to participate in the classroom as volunteers. The teacher should have excellent skills at working with adults as well as with children. The teacher of the multihandicapped must take a strong position of leadership in designing and coordinating the educational services to be provided. The related services should always be provided so that the instructor is kept constantly abreast of the specifics of the program and can assure the classroom and home the continuity of the program. Interdisciplinary staffings should be conducted periodically to discuss progress. These meetings need focus and direction and should be conducted by the teacher or the direct supervisor in order to assure the results have classroom applicability.

The team leader competency, which is forced upon the teacher, comes in addition to those resulting from the needs of each child in the class. Many of these needs may be in areas where a teacher has had little specific training. It is essential that teachers acknowledge their strengths as well as their weaknesses in order that consultative assistance may be provided where necessary. Teachers need to acknowledge their strengths in order to offset the inevitable disappointments with the long list of successes. Such balance is important to work at in order to reduce frustration and avoid the high teacher fatigue rate characteristic in programs for the severely and profoundly handicapped. Poor multi-factored evaluations or reports will provide little support to the teacher. The design of the physical space, of the emotional environment, and of the schedule for each instructional assistant should find their basis in the multi-factored evaluation data provided as well as the personality and additional data offered by the current teacher.

Many factors will effect the success or failure of attempts to implement the annual goals and short-term instructional objectives contained in the IEP. One of the keys to long-term success is long-range planning based on effective interagency coordination. In addition to the public schools, there are many other agencies involved with the early childhood identification, evaluation, and educational programs for multi-handicapped children and their families. Input from these agencies must of necessity be successfully coordinated by the public schools who will eventually assume the responsibility to make an educational placement. At the other end of the special education continuum are those agencies dealing with the provision of rehabilitation training and alternative residential service providers. These agencies should begin to become involved with the family and school in planning for the child's future, and this should take place around the child's sixteenth birthday. Diagnostic vocational assessments should be provided by rehabilitation specialists, and suggestions should be made relative to the appropriate goals and objectives to consider. Information may also be provided about the continuum of work alternatives available in the community for the multi-handicapped and the requirements necessary for successful functioning in each available alternative.

Parents should be asked if they would like to meet and discuss the continuum of residential options available for their child upon completion of school. They are the primary decision-makers in instances where the student is unable to express meaningful, personal preferences about where to live. Educators can assist parents to come into contact with other parents who have had to make a variety of placement decisions and are willing to share both the feelings and experiences they have had in seeking the options related to those decisions. Parents should also be given access to the variety of professionals who would assist them in finding a least restrictive residential placement. The availability of a variety of acceptable alternative residential options is essential to the successful continuation of learning as an adult. It is important to note that the educator acts more as a resource in making others available to help evaluate the needs of the student and is not to be viewed as the primary evaluation resource in this area.

The assessment and placement of a preschool child with multi-handicaps is a commitment to providing an appropriate continuum of services until the responsibility of special education ends at age twenty-two or until the completion of the school program before this age. It will often be appropriate to have various agencies and professionals involved in some stages of development and not in others. To assume the attitude that the future will take care of itself, or that today's educational answers are going to be in line with tomorrow's educational needs, is a dangerously inappropriate posture. The section of the IEP that requires those writing it to predict the anticipated duration that special education services are likely to be needed should be a painful reminder of the need for long-term planning and for coordination of services for the multi-handicapped. Appropriate program options must be identified or developed from early childhood through the post-secondary level to provide the training that will be required.

The relationship between assessment and program implementation is not one that results from the perfunctory completion of ten easy rules. It is the result of a delicately designed, child centered, interpersonal, and professional process requiring openness, realism, long-term planning, and coordination between the many persons who will be involved.

ISSUES AND PROBLEMS

Many of the issues and problems experienced by educators specifically designated as serving the multi-handicapped are shared by professionals in the special education programs for the deaf, the visually handicapped, the moderately, severely, and profoundly mentally retarded, and the orthopedic and other health impaired. The following list of concerns briefly states some of the current issues raised by those operating such programs. Items discussed are related to assessment, placement, implementation, and the law.

1. There are transportation problems inherent in the operation of any educational program for a population with an extremely low incidence figure. How far is too far to travel? How long is too long to sit? How appropriate is it to transport multi-physically handicapped students in equipment not appropriately designed or adapted to meet their needs? How expensive is it, and who will pay the bill for appropriate

transportation?

The school district is responsible to provide a free and appropriate form of transportation for each handicapped child. What is appropriate? The definition of appropriate transportation services should be determined by the group of persons writing the IEP. Transportation services are considered related services. It is one of the many services that may be provided to assist a child to benefit from special education. What may be an appropriate time on the bus, or an appropriate type of vehicle at one point, may not be appropriate at another point in the school carrier. The effect of excessive travel time or inappropriate posture while being transported can be significant and may relate directly to the possibilities for successful classroom intervention. Discussion about the appropriateness of an issue related to transportation is an acceptable reason to request a periodic review of the IEP.

In many states, parents may be asked if they would like to transport their own handicapped child to school. In certain instances the parents may choose not to do so as the ultimate responsibility for providing this service lies with the local school districts. If parents do transport their child, they should not be asked to provide this service at a cost less than that which they incur. No matter what is decided to be the right form of transportation, the assessment information, particularly that which relates to the stamina and physical nature of a child's handicaps, should be considered.

2. The duration of the school day, and the school year, are often issues in the multi-handicapped program. The school instructional day should never summarily be diminished from that offered to all other students in the system. The child with multi-handicaps should not have the instructional day diminished as a result of extensive travel. The teaching day is often cut short because the buses arrive late and/or are scheduled to leave school early, reducing the school day as much as one to one and one-half hours per day. The only instance where a handicapped child's school day should be less than the average day is when the IEP specifically calls for a reduced day. Decisions of this nature are usually made based on classroom observation, the observation of parents, and interpretation of

medical information and other assessment data.

There are many persons who would argue that most children with multi-handicaps could benefit from an extended school year program. There are many who consider the three-month summer break too long and too costly because of the skills the students may lose and the consequent retraining they will need before the new progress can be pursued in the fall. However, in the absence of specialized legislation authorizing school districts to expend public funds to operate summer programs, many such programs have not been created. Additionally, in a time when local taxpayers are reluctant to provide enough tax support to keep the basic operation of the regular school program alive; in a time when a state legislators sense the political necessity to levy no further taxes; and in a time when the recent federal and state mandates to serve all handicapped children have doubled the services and programs available to the handicapped population without providing the full funding necessary; it is realistically impossible to expect immediate political enthusiasm or action. There are states that offer extended school year programs for those with multi-handicaps, but most do not. There are states where extended programs currently operating are in danger of being cut out because they are not mandated, and money is becoming increasingly difficult to raise. It looks as though the provision of free summer programs for handicapped children in the immediate future will continue to be relegated predominantly to special grants from funds other than those provided by the public schools unless the due process and legal actions pending on this issue require the provision of an extended school year. (The *Armstrong* v. *Kline* case in Pennsylvania has recently been heard in a federal district court. The ruling states that the school district must fund summer education for those handicapped children who show that an interruption of schooling would be detrimental to their progress. Pennsylvania has appealed this decision.)

3. The rapid turnover in staff associated with programs educating children with severe handicaps is of great concern to those who would build programs with stability and continuity. The excessive need to retrain persons to the peculiar characteristics of the population is also a source of disillusionment to

many supervisors and administrators. Too many teachers burn out. Factors related to teacher fatigue include service training, insufficient descriptive assessment information, and sparse curriculum resources.

4. There will inevitably be an age beyond which the local school district will assume no further responsibility for the education of a handicapped person. There is no effective requirement that agencies such as education and rehabilitation must coordinate their evaluation and programming services to assure continuity from the special education system into the rehabilitation service agency upon leaving school. This is the ultimate in poor planning! It is certainly one of the most frustrating situations the parents of a severely handicapped adult can experience in their struggle to assure that the services necessary to provide lifelong help and support to the multi-handicapped are maintained. Too often it is the lack of good union between the education, rehabilitation, and residential service providers, combined with the few options available to parents in the residential and rehabilitation areas, that have forced the excessive and unnecessary institutionalization of many multi-handicapped adults.

Special educators cannot solve the inadequate funding of the legislation necessary to create stronger rehabilitation and residential service continuums; however, they can improve their secondary evaluation and programming efforts to include the training of the necessary habits and skills to function in a variety of work and home settings. To assess and train more effectively in these two areas two parties will have to be called upon much more to provide direct consultation and evaluation resources during the high school years. Rehabilitation evaluators and parents need to be much more involved in the areas of work and domestic skills as well as in the design of secondary multi-factored evaluation and special education programs. The spirit of recent cooperative letters of agreement between the federal agencies with responsibility for vocational education, special education, and rehabilitation services and of the recently passed P.L. 95-602 will have to filter down to the local level and be translated into local cooperative policies and procedures. When and if this happens, the necessary transition from youth to adulthood, and from education to the many agencies coordinating adult services for the multi-handicapped, can be improved.

5. The tremendous need to expand services and programs available for those with multi-handicaps, as provided for in P.L. 94-142, and as necessitated by the many assessed needs of the multi-handicapped, has created many due process hearings. While some due process cases are concerned with such general issues as summer programming, private school placement, placement in segregated facilities, and others, there are many more dealing with much more local and child-specific issues. These issues include decisions to be made about the appropriateness of evaluation data used, a pending placement decision, and the special education and related services currently identified on, or omitted from, the IEP. In this latter group of locally created and resolvable issues, there are many concerns for educators related to and resulting from the collection and interpretation of child assessment data.

The resolution of many cases is unduly influenced by the tremendous cost to the local school district of entering into a due process hearing. Some school districts are unwilling and unable to pursue their professional beliefs about a particular case merely because of the thousands of dollars they might have to expend to elucidate them. The use of mediation techniques might be helpful in these instances if the parents are willing to enter into discussions with a district short of a due process hearing. These mediation techniques are referred to in Section 121a.506 *Comment*, of the Federal Rules and Regulations:

> *Comment*: Many states have pointed to the success of using mediation as an intervening step prior to conducting a formal due process hearing. Although the process of mediation is not required by the statute or these regulations, an agency may wish to suggest mediation in disputes concerning the identification, evaluation, and educational placement of handicapped children, and the provision of a free appropriate public education to those children. Mediations have been conducted by members of state educational agencies or local educational agency personnel who were not previously involved in the particular case. In many cases, mediation leads to resolution of differences between parents and agencies

without the development of an adversarial relationship and
with minimal emotional stress. However, mediation may not
be used to deny or delay a parent's rights under this subpart.

It would appear that more attempts by states and school
districts to create and use mediation mechanisms would bring
about a less expensive and more efficient way to deal with local
problems, in a fair and objective fashion. Parents or agencies
may still choose to request a due process hearing and avoid any
mediation activities. Examples of mediation techniques might
include an administrative review with the local superintendent
wherein the superintendent attempts to serve as an arbitrator in
the dispute. Another example is the use of State Department of
Special Education staff as mediators between agencies or between agencies and parents. Finally, local and state level strategies, to effectively receive and follow up on parental complaint,
also helps to resolve problems related to the assessment and
placement process as quickly as possible and at the lowest level
of escalation within the due process system.

The purpose of the due process procedures related to impartial hearings is to provide a format for assuring that decisions
are made in the best interests of children. The cost of these
hearings alone may be a prohibitive factor for some school
districts and may cause them to compromise in a direction not
in the best interests of the child in order to avoid the expense.
The clear need for the due process hearing option is uncontes-
table. Both parents and local agencies, however, need several
means of interfacing available to them prior to due process.
These options can result in an equitable solution with little or
no additional expense. The question is whether the cost of the
due process hearing is prohibitive as a decision-making tool for
a school district.

6. In addition to the local school district, many individuals
and groups have taken on the role of providing parents and
professionals with technical information and advocacy services.
Providing parents with a working understanding of their rights
and encouraging them to exercise their role as informed con-
sumers of education is a formidable task. Too often, in the past,
educators have influenced many parents with a "take it or leave
it" attitude about the special education services and programs

provided. Until P.L. 94-142 guaranteed a free and just education to all handicapped children, and until the due process system was provided for those who would challenge the quality of the measures being taken to educate a handicapped child, parents had little recourse. Today's schools are constantly challenged to be both the provider of services and a primary advocate for the children's special education needs. This dual role cannot always be effectively implemented. The services of advocates are often necessary to challenge the schools to improve services and to better educate parents concerning their rights. The issues that emerge when trying to deliver free and just education to multi-handicapped children have resulted in many due process hearings and have involved many advocates and advocacy groups.

The history of due process hearings within each state and across the nation, as well as the legal decisions that have resulted from the appeals of many of these hearings, are a source of much study and influence on current and future programs for the severely handicapped. Advocates are providing a necessary catalyst for change in issues affecting as few as one child and in issues affecting large numbers of handicapped children. They are a necessary and effective source of support to parents who find they have reached an impasse with their local school district.

The evaluation process is the most significant aspect of the pre-placement procedures. It will effect the need for, the direction of, and the outcome of any due process proceedings. Issues related to the appropriateness and extensiveness of existing evaluations, the need for independent evaluations, the appropriateness of the activities conducted to complete the prior notice requirements of Sections 121a.504 and 121a.505, and issues related to the determination of students as handicapped, are all essentially evaluation issues. Special educators can no longer limit the evaluation and services to those which they themselves are capable of helping..Outside help will be needed. Every child suspected of being handicapped has to be assessed in all areas related to the suspected disability.

Advocates are often very welcome and helpful partners in assuring the delivery of appropriate special education services.

Often they will not be directly embroiled in the early stages of the conflict. They offer more of a public forum for the resolution of problems. The entry of an advocate, even at the level of a phone call, may be all that it takes to assist program implementors and/or parents to overcome the roadblocks to the full implementation of an appropriate program. There are other instances when an advocate's involvement creates unnecessary expectations which exceed the realistic needs of the child and the circumstances. In these instances, their work hinders the delivery of an appropriate program.

The unrealistic match of mandates and available money, the periodically insufficient activities of local school districts on behalf of children suspected of having handicaps, and the existence of the procedural safeguards system will support the need for advocacy services for some time to come.

7. The time required to manage the child information management systems, and the interdisciplinary coordination of personnel involved in the initial evaluations, the periodic reviews, the three-year reevaluations, and the procedural safeguard activities is creating a problem of crisis proportions. All of these evaluation activities are appropriate and essential. They require extensive documentation, an efficient recordkeeping system, and a management and planning system capable of assisting evaluation personnel in monitoring the status of many handicapped children who are at different steps in the evaluation, placement, and reevaluation cycle.

The role of the school psychologist, to whom much of the long-term management of this system generally falls, is further complicated by the excellent requirement that evaluations must be conducted by more than one person from more than one discipline. School principals and guidance counselors are also pressed into serving as case managers for parts or all of the evaluation and case management continuum. The involvement of these persons is often essential but further taxes the existing manpower available to provide the multitude of services necessary in the schools. The primary evaluators themselves are often so caught up in conducting initial and reevaluation activities that the frequently necessary follow-up observations, consultative services, and sometimes even the quality of the written evaluation reports, suffer. The extended responsibilities of evaluators and administrators as a result of the requirement of P.L. 94-142 will either result in the eventual hiring of new staff or in the likelihood of diminished services offered in other areas by these individuals. The resentment generated and the services lost, if the latter alternative is the only available choice, would be a significant and an unfortunate byproduct of offering evaluation and placement services in compliance with the law.

8. What is it like to have a child with multi-handicaps? Professional evaluators and special educators should be familiar with the literature in this area. They should also consider it essential to find out the unique circumstances and feelings of each family with whom they work. The educational and other decisions made by the parents of children with multi-handicaps are made with the history of their experiences with medical and educational personnel in mind. The decisions will be made based on the unique circumstances and needs of their family unit. They will be made with much consideration given to the feelings, as well as to the consideration of the facts involved. This is not to say that the special educator either desires to provide, or is qualified to provide, family psychological therapy services. Neither does this suggest that parents are in need of, or desire these services. The parents of any child should be treated holistically, or as integrated personalities, by each person who provides them services. The educator who provides only diagnostic "facts" and "intervention strategies," however appropriate, without attempting to understand the perspective and needs of those parents who are listening, is blazing a personally "safe" but less than effective educational trail for the child involved. It is not uncommon for this exclusive emphasis on the immediate discovery of remediation strategies and diagnostic labels to significantly reduce the effectiveness of the multi-factored evaluation process.

9. There are many publicly and privately owned residential facilities for children with multi-handicaps. These facilities are all located within the boundaries of local school districts which, according to Section 121a.324, have the responsibility to provide the following assurances:

A local educational agency may use funds provided under

Part B of the Act for second priority children if it provides assurance satisfactory to the state educational agency in its application (or an amendment to this application);

(a) That all first priority children have a free appropriate public education available to them;

(b) That the local educational agency has a system for the identification, location, and evaluation of handicapped children, as described in its application; and

(c) That whenever a first priority child is identified, located, and evaluated, the local educational agency makes available a free, appropriate public education to the child.

Each of these local school districts also has the responsibility to make available an appropriate special education program in the least restrictive alternative as required in Section 121a.550, and even more specifically, in the comment following Section 121a.554, stating:

Comment: Under section 612(5)(B) of the statute the requirement to educate handicapped children with nonhandicapped children also applies to children in public and private institutions or other care facilities. Each state educational agency must insure that each applicable agency and institution in the state implements this requirement. Regardless of other reasons for institutional placement, no child in an institution who is capable of education in a regular public school setting may be denied access to an education in that setting.

There are extensive problems experienced by small school districts confronted with the challenge to identify, evaluate, and make available an appropriate special education program to the many children with multi-handicaps who might reside in a facility within their boundaries. The location of the whereabouts of the parents or guardians is cumbersome and sometimes impossible without the aid of the courts. Most of the students in the facility are likely to have been placed from out of the district or even from out of the state. This makes the procedural safeguard section of the evaluation process excessively time consuming. The designation of each identified student's school district of legal residence is another problem. This depends much on the results obtained when trying to identify the whereabouts of parents and guardians and will

then involve offering a special education program to the school
district of legal residence for them to make a placement in. The
school district of residence either makes the suggested placement, goes to due process to challenge the suggested placement,
or provides an appropriate program themselves.

What are the financial arrangements and problems? There is
a great likelihood that there will be costs well over the sending
districts regular tuition rate because of the adaptive equipment
and transportation necessary, the low pupil teacher ratio, and
the many related services that are customarily needed. Sometimes students are placed from out of the state, and there are
special financial circumstances which may require reimburse-
ment for all costs incurred because state funds may not be
legally spent for legal residents of other states.

Housing the special education teachers and classes may be a
problem. The school district may not have enough available
empty classroom space to provide housing for a large newly
identified group of multi-handicapped students. Students may
be unable to be appropriately transported to an educational
setting outside of the residential facility due to medical reasons.

These and other issues combine to create problems for the
local school district that happens to have a residential facility
serving the multi-handicapped within its boundary. It is entirely possible that not one child housed in the facility is a
child whose school district of legal residence is the community
in which the facility is housed. Finally, the developmental
levels of many of the children needing special education services are frequently at the profound level which more than
likely will require the district to obtain extensive assistance in
providing useful and appropriate multi-factored evaluations.

10. Each state agency has the responsibility to evaluate and
monitor the activities of all public agencies within the state
relative to their compliance with federal and state mandates,
according to Sections 121a.600-602. State education agencies
must develop policies and procedures to conduct these responsibilities. To the extent that these monitoring procedures are
very specific, and are communicated in writing to those agencies who are to be reviewed, they can assist education agencies
to self-monitor their compliance with the law. State agency

staff, on official reviews, or local educators conducting self-monitoring reviews of evaluation-related requirements, should follow the order in which activities logically occur. Answers to all questions about requirements should be substantiated in the educational records reviewed. The purpose of this review should go beyond compliance monitoring. It should seek to identify whether there is continuity between the assessment data obtained, the placement decisions made, and the nature of the IEP that is written. Efforts should also be made to identify the manner and the extent to which parents are presented with their rights and included in the IEP development process. The most significant impact of the monitoring process is its ability to provide agencies with personalized technical assistance. Most special educators are making extensive efforts to comply with the rash of new special education regulations resulting from P.L. 94-142. They deserve a monitoring procedure that both challenges and assists them to design special education programs that are in full compliance with the law. As the guesswork surrounding what is required in special education programs that comply with the law begins to lift, so should the mystery about how to design such programs.

11. Who runs special education? Do children's and parents' needs dictate everything that takes place? Do special education personnel and their professional organizations? Do local and state boards of education? Do state and federal agency bureaucrats decide much of what goes on? Do the courts, or do politicians? The answer to the question about who is shaping the future of special education is extremely important. The answer sheds much light on what strategies persons with multi-handicaps, or their advocates, will need to employ to achieve their full educational potential.

The traditional school used to be more controlled by its local school board, its superintendent, and all of the parental, community, and professional pressure groups that surrounded it. Special education programs have always been much influenced by state policies and standards, but historically these standards have never been as detailed or comprehensive or as well enforced as recent legislation requires them to be.

Politicians, through increased legislative activity which has often resulted from landmark court cases, are moving more and more to the fore. Locating the money necessary to provide the services for the multi-handicapped is the major remaining hurdle to be overcome. Sections 121a.301 and 121a.600 of P.L. 94-142 in Federal Rules and Regulations clearly indicate that the school district with responsibility for making the special education program placement, and ultimately the state education agency, are responsible to assure that the special education and related services necessary are provided. There is no legal way for a school district to cite lack of funds in refusing to provide special education services for a child. If legislators at the federal and state levels do not more fully fund the special education programs they have mandated, school personnel will be further required to divide their failing local resources.

CONCLUSION

No system of effectively evaluating and educating children with multi-handicaps will function to its capacity without the support of parents; without the professional and creative efforts of evaluators, teachers, and administrators; and without the necessary authorization and funding. The recent passage of P.L. 94-142 and the dissemination and implementation of the regulations resulting from that bill have done much to further delineate and assure that each handicapped child will receive a free and appropriate public education. This law and the associated regulations require many more assurances of detailed compliance at the local and state level than have been required in the past. Compliance with this law is also tied directly to the allocation of federal funds to each school district. There is no doubt that this bill has resulted in increased federal control over programs for the handicapped.

Are the issues over which the bill has exercised control necessary ones? Most have no trouble answering that the philosophical issues raised in the Education for All Handicapped Childrens Act of 1975 are both necessary and helpful. What is this law's impact on the evaluation process itself? The process is now much more comprehensive and detailed than at any other time in the past. The problems related to the assessment of the multi-handicapped that have resulted from the passage, implementation, and partial funding of this bill are more the result of the unique needs and circumstances of the multi-handicapped child than those related to the legislation itself.

The successful integration of the legislative mandates into the assessment process, the determination of a suitable special education program for each identified handicapped child, the design of appropriate classroom organization, and the resolution of all the issues and problems mentioned in this chapter will combine to meet the needs of the multi-handicapped if the attitudes of professionals and parents do not place arbitrary limits on their realistic capabilities and needs. The evaluation team that believes in the dignity and potential to be discovered in each child, and that works with the family to create a challenging and realistic set of educational goals and objectives, will have accomplished most of the intent of the law. Recent efforts to become familiar with and to implement the detailed procedural requirements of the law may have temporarily led some professionals to attend more to their new administrative environment than to the persons this environment is designed to help serve. The process of change is often confusing and it leads many to yearn for "the good old days." The future of assessment, however, will become less cumbersome as refinement of the administrative requirements makes them more manageable and as familiarity with them brings increased efficiency and confidence.

REFERENCES

Brown, L.; Nietupski, J.; and Hamre-Nietupski, S. The criterion of ultimate functioning and public school services for severely handicapped students. In Brown, L.; Certo, N.; and Crowner, T. (Eds,): *Papers and Programs Related to Public School Services for Secondary — Age Severely Handicapped Students.* Madison, Wisconsin, Madison Metropolitan School District, 1976, vol. I, part I. (Republished: *Hey, Don't Forget About Me: New Directions for Serving the Severely Handicapped.* Reston, Virginia, Coun Exc Child, 1976, pp. 2-15.
"The Federal Education for All Handicapped Children Act (P.L. 94-142)." Signed, November 29, 1975. Reston, Virginia, Coun Exc Child, 1976.
"Final Regulations: Implementation of Part B of the Education of the Handicapped Act," effective October, 1977. U.S. Office of Education,

Department of Health, Education, and Welfare. U.S. Govt. Print., Washington, D.C.

"Planning Instruction for the Severely Handicapped," North Carolina Department of Public Instruction, V, 1978. Division of Exceptional Children.

"Program Review and Evaluation Procedures for Special Education," Ohio Department of Education. July, 1978.

Writer, Jan. "The Design of Instructional Programs for Severely Handicapped Students," a paper in *Educational Methods for Deaf-Blind and Severely Handicapped Students.* Texas Education Agency, January 1979, vol. 1, pp. 16-40.

CHAPTER TWO

EDUCATORS' CONSIDERATIONS IN ESTABLISHING ASSESSMENT PROGRAMS FOR SEVERE/MULTIPLE UNITS

JOSEPH MURRAY, PH.D.

AGAIN, as it has happened so often in the history of special education, legislation prompted by the perceived needs of parents, interest groups, and educators has spawned a major change in the configuration of special education programming. Public law 94-142 has clearly delineated responsibilities of educators relevant to the education of children with special needs by insuring such actions as identification of *all* handicapped children and the placement of these children into the least restrictive environment. This legislation requires that each state not only establish a goal of full service for handicapped children presently being educationally provided for, but also mandates that each state establish priorities for serving those youngsters who are currently unserved.

The establishment in 1975 of P.L. 94-142 caused many states to look closely at their special education programming and to rethink along the lines of how best to meet its dictates. Public law 93-380 adopted on August 21, 1974 had given direction to massive change in special education programming; now P.L. 94-142 has modified and refined that law and, most importantly, has demonstrated that the dollars would be available to facilitate the programming. Guided by 93-380, many state boards of education adopted a set of program standards for what was to become an integral part of the plan to help provide full service programming standards for the implementation of programs to serve heretofore unserved or inappropriately served handicapped children. One of the best and yet not atypical examples of how legislation effected a change in special education programming can be found in the state of Ohio. The

Division of Special Education there has markedly increased the number of severe and/or multi-handicapped units in an attempt to provide a free and appropriate education for all. As will be described later, the severe and/or multi-handicapped units are designed to provide education and training for youngsters having a variety of handicapping conditions. The increase in the number of severe and/or multiple units since 1974 has been considerable as indicated by the following figures and represents the national trend in providing education for multi-handicapped children:

School Year	Number of Multi-handicapped Units
1974-75	25
1975-76	47
1976-77	92
1977-78	134
1978-79	200

Many states have maintained special education programs for the retarded, for the learning disabled, the behaviorally disordered, and other long-recognized handicaps. Not specifically and effectively provided for, however, were youngsters having multi-handicaps, often victimized by a combination of vision impairment, hearing impairment, different types of aphasia, physical and brain anomalies or autisticlike behaviors. These youngsters constitute the type of child qualifying for the severe/multi-handicapped units. Often pervasive throughout these disorders is a concomitant of emotional, behavioral, familial, and psychological problems. Recognition of youngsters possessing these multiple disorders has dictated the need for a different approach to assessment and different educational/ training programs for this type of child.

With the trend toward continued development of programs to serve the multi-handicapped, educators have realized that traditionally used diagnostic and programming efforts were not providing functional diagnostic information to teachers, aids, and others who worked with multi-handicapped children. The mid-to-late 70s has seen much more emphasis on functional diagnosis and programming and a movement away from diagnosing children as "statistical entities" and providing these entities with cookbook remedial programs.

Educators have realized the importance of developing assessment methods that allow for comprehensive description of children across all domains, and it has been recognized that the findings derived from the individual assessment must be tied-in with meaningful prescriptive programming for the child.

With the help of a title VI-D grant, awarded by the Division of Special Education in Ohio and with further assistance offered by a grant from Kent State University in Ohio, the subject of educating multi-handicapped youngsters was studied over a period of four years. Teachers and other educators working with this type of youngster were brought together for the purpose of furthering understanding of the many issues related to assessment and programming for these types of handicaps. Reported in the following pages of this chapter is information shared by those educators on the "firing line" who dealt with issues related to the broader concept of the multi-handicapped child and the more specific topic of diagnosis of this type of child.

Who is the multi-handicapped child? How do educators describe the type of child for whom special non-normative assessment and individualized programming must be afforded? The following characteristics represent the consensus of thought arrived at by over fifty special educators in Ohio in answering the aforementioned questions:

1. Severe and/or multi-handicapped children frequently have some type of receptive or expressive language disorder.
2. Many manifest severe behavioral disorder(s).
3. Most do not have observable physical anomalies.
4. Many youngsters have autistic characteristics such as language disorders and a propensity for perseverative behaviors, echolalia, ritualistic behavior, self-destructive behavior, and extremely withdrawn behavior.
5. Evidence exists to suggest that the child cannot properly be accommodated in any existing special education program.
6. Multi-handicapped youngsters often have a developmental

age of as low as one month. These types of handicaps carry with them a wide range of disabilities and great severity of functional disability making even more important the concept of functional, individualized assessment. This type of disability also introduces the element of diagnosing for "training" purposes as well as diagnosing for educational purposes.

The multi-handicapped child with his mild-to-severe deficiencies in multiple domains often is unable to be assessed using typical normative instrumentation and practices. Educators working on a daily basis with multi-handicapped children know this and stress a number of points related to assessment which psychologists, special educators, and others working with the multi-handicapped need to know.

INDIVIDUAL CHILDREN AS ENTITIES UNTO THEMSELVES

One overriding theme came from discussing with teachers of the multi-handicapped what they believed to be important in the assessment process. Each child is different, and it should be the goal of the assessment process to clearly describe the child as an *entity* unto him or herself (Murray 1979). Using the five basic domains of motor, cognition, social/emotional, language, and achievement, the end result of the assessment should describe children in terms of their strengths and weaknesses with attention being given to developmental levels across all domains. Teachers uniformly minimize the importance of standardized assessment devices, such as the Wechsler Intelligence Test for Children (revised) and the Stanford-Binet, opting instead for criterion-referenced instrumentation that would functionally describe the child. As a thought to those professionals who might be involved in establishing an assessment program for multi-handicapped youngsters, it should be pointed out that "parts" of standardized tests might be considered for usage in an attempt to more fully complete the diagnostic "picture" of a multi-handicapped child. As an example, Wechsler subtests, such as block designs or mazes, might be used to gain information about a child's abstract reasoning capability or about his reflectivity capacity in problem solving. No other parts of the Wechsler would be used. In addition to using parts of standardized tests in an assessment battery, entire specialized tests such as the Columbia Test of Mental Maturity or the Leiter International Performance Scale might be used with a child having a severe speech impairment. This would give the teacher a better understanding of the child's cognitive level, and this information could be coupled with the less formal criterion-referenced material, again, for the purpose of gaining a more complete picture of the child.

THE CONCEPT OF ONGOING DIAGNOSIS

Educators and, in particular, psychologists have become oriented to a one-time assessment of children which has typically generated a statistical description to the exclusion of a more meaningful (functional) description of a child. Legislation such as P.L. 94-142 as well as the unique characteristics of the multi-handicapped child, which make meaningless normative assessment in many cases, have been responsible for the development of the concept of ongoing diagnosis. In some instances, the term "diagnostic classroom" has been used in describing classes for the multi-handicapped, which suggests that gaining a functional understanding of a multi-handicapped child is and has to be an ongoing process. Because of the uniqueness and multiplicity of the handicaps possessed by multi-handicapped youngsters, the need for an intensive and comprehensive ongoing assessment is of paramount importance.

In order to effect a comprehensive assessment of youngsters entering and attending classes for the multi-handicapped, provisions should be made for conducting a multi-factored evaluation using an interdisciplinary approach. Descriptive evaluation data should be compiled from as many of the following areas as deemed necessary for determining the child's educational performance including his learning characteristics and his unique educational needs: medical history, educational and developmental history, personal/social/emotional functioning, cognitive functioning, academic functioning, vocational/occupational needs, communication skills, gross/fine/sensory motor skills, and adaptive behavior. The compilation of this data will require not only the input from parents and teachers, but may also require the services of orthopedic, physical, vision, hearing, language, speech, medical specialists, and psychologists.

In addition to the interdisciplinary approach, all of these components should be considered as vital to a complete assessment program.

NON-NORMATIVE ASSESSMENT

The domains of fine and gross motor, cognition, language, self-help skills, academic level, social adaptability, and possibly vocational as well should constitute the core of the assessment. Unlike traditional approaches, assessment of the multi-handicapped has been found to be most effective when the following principles are adhered to (Murray 1979).

Functional, descriptive, and when possible, normative assessment should be conducted, e.g. describe the child while at the same time obtaining developmental levels on given domains. The advantage of determining initial developmental levels can be seen when reevaluation is necessary. To facilitate assessment and to insure a compilation of knowledge across all applicable domains, certain functional assessment instruments have been developed. A complete listing of these instruments listed by type of handicap can be found later in this book.

Many teachers have found television tapes to be helpful in assessing behavioral and motor change. Often, weekly or monthly changes are so subtle that persons working with the child daily do not perceive them. Television tapes provide the opportunity to contrast behavior over time and also permit more objective assessment since tapes can be replayed constantly. Reliability in terms of base-line data and measuring intervention effects can be improved by the use of television.

OBSERVATION OF THE CHILD

Informal observation in a setting familiar to the child will give the examiner an opportunity to better understand how the child has learned to adapt to his immediate environment. It is generally better to see the child in an environment familiar to him so that the assessment is not confused by the child's inability to adapt to new situations. The more handicapped the child is, the more he is likely to have had limited social experiences and limited ability to accommodate new situations and people.

During the informal observation period, an examiner who is relatively unfamiliar with a certain type of child will have an opportunity to become accustomed to the qualities of the particular handicap. An important factor that is infrequently discussed involves many examiners' unfamiliarity and resulting discomfort with certain types of handicapping conditions. By allowing for an informal interview and observation period, the examiner can "ease into" an evaluation in a more comfortable manner rather than being imposed upon by the necessity for immediate involvement with a formal diagnostic assessment. The observation period will also provide for the examiner an opportunity to answer many of the questions on formal instrumentation such as the screening checklist, the interview form, and the medical/developmental history.

Another consideration involves permitting the *parent* to observe the evaluator's interactions with the child. This will permit the evaluator to ask whether or not the child is responding in a typical manner or if there are things the child usually does but is not doing at the present time. Parent input at this time can also help parents to focus more carefully on their child's assets and limitations. This is particularly important if there is a discrepancy between the parent's perceptions of their child and what the evaluator observes. If the evaluation process is open at least in part to the parent's view, the basis of recommendations is more likely to be understood and follow through is more likely to occur. The philosophy is quite unlike that of many adherants to strict standardization, usually seen in normative testing, but does allow for a more functional description of the child.

During the observation period, the evaluator has an opportunity to make judgments regarding the child's sensory and/or response capabilities and limitations. Using the various domains as a frame of reference, actual observations can be made.

During this time, situations can be set up to assess specific capabilities. Some examples follow (Matey 1975):

1. Fine and gross motor skills can be observed by having the child play with toys and other materials. If the child is seen in the home, his parents can be asked to bring out his favorite toys; if he is in a familiar setting, materials with which the child is familiar can be chosen. For example, it is important to determine how a child can grasp and place objects, and this can be assessed by using puzzles, peg-boards, balls, form boards, or a paper and pencil. If the child needs assistance in performing motor tasks, the degree of assistance should be noted.

2. Gross social relating skills can be best assessed in the informal assessment. The evaluator should observe whether the child establishes eye contact, looks up for feedback as to the correctness of a response, or ignores others. The evaluator can determine how well the child responds to direction from an adult by giving simple commands and observing how well the child responds. Odd mannerisms and unusual preoccupations, e.g. arm-flapping, finger-flicking, or string-twirling and the conditions under which they occur can be noted. The evaluator can assess the child's readiness for a more formal school program by trying to stimulate such an experience; this can be done by structuring a situation in which the child is sitting down at a table while various tasks are presented with accompanying demands. Various reinforcers can also be attempted and their effectiveness determined.

3. Self-care can be assessed to the extent that the examiner has time and opportunities occur. Parent reports can be checked in the areas of relative dependence in toileting, eating, and dressing. Again it should be mentioned that the assessor of the child who is experienced in interviewing can fill in many of the questions asked on the formal assessment devices by closely observing the child within his environment.

4. Communication skills are often impaired in handicapped children. It is good to record a sample of each child's expressive communication skills and to observe how well

the child responds to others' attempts to communicate. This may begin on a basic level with a determination of whether or not the child turns when someone calls his name or whether he points toward something he wants. Often, communication can be prompted by creating a need, e.g. taking a desired object from the child. Normally, however, if given an unstructured play situation in a familiar environment, even children with communication handicaps will express themselves to the extent that they are able.

5. Cognitive and academic skills can be assessed informally by presenting various tasks in a playlike manner. The child's facility with pre-academic skills e.g. puzzles, color and shape discrimination, may overlap with other areas, e.g. motor assessment, but also included may be skills more readily classified as cognitively based. The evaluator can present picture books, counting tasks, simple reading exercises, and the like to determine the child's relative readiness for academic instruction.

In summary, observational procedures can yield much information about a child and can form the basis upon which selection of formal assessment tools can be made. A good observational session will minimize the likelihood that time will be spent on assessment procedures that are inappropriate for a particular child.

ASSESSMENT BY PHYSICIAN

Teachers and educators whom we interviewed that were affiliated with multi-handicapped classes almost uniformly reported the need for having medical evaluation available for all children. They also suggested the need for better communication between the physician and the teaching staff. Many multi-handicapped youngsters have physiologically based disorders. The medical component of the assessment of multi-handicapped youngsters should provide the teacher and her staff with an understanding of the disorder and its ramifications plus an awareness of her role in coping with that disorder in the classroom. Teachers typically reported that the medical aspect of the assessment program was the weakest in terms of the awareness and the help which it afforded them in providing for the child. An ideal assessment program, it was suggested, would provide a written, understandable, and educationally relevant medical report followed by a period of consultation with the physician in which educators could ask meaningful and necessary questions to the physician about specific children. This assessment-related concept was felt to be so important by teachers that many suggested building funds into the assessment program to allow for medical assessment and consultation.

MEDICAL/DEVELOPMENTAL ASSESSMENT

A comprehensive medical/developmental history taken from the parents in addition to information received from a physician can help to fill in the assessment picture. It helps to facilitate interaction and communication between parent and professional and, most importantly, gives vital information related to the child's historical development to date. There are a number of developmental interview forms on the market, all of which seem to have the following basic components: family history, gestational and perinatal history, developmental history (questions related to the attainment of developmental milestones such as when the chid first stood, walked, and used phrases). Past medical history, psychosocial history (questions related to sibling relations, feeding problems, sleep problems, activity level, the child's affective characteristics, and his/her likes and dislikes), and educational history are important components found on most interview forms. While medical/developmental information forms are often felt to lack reliability, they can add much to the total assessment findings and are often overlooked when establishing an assessment program for the multiply handicapped. The following medical/developmental history, adapted from an instrument developed by CIBA Pharmaceutical Company, Summit, New Jersey, illustrates the information areas and the types of questions which should be asked to gain information about a child's medical/developmental history.

Table 2-I

MEDICAL/DEVELOPMENTAL HISTORY

Date
_____

Name of Patient
_____

FAMILY HISTORY

1. What are the ages of both parents?

2. What is their occupation or past occupations?

3. What is the current health status of both parents?

4. What past health problems have they experienced?

5. What is the nature of the family constellation?

6. What other pregnancies did the mother have?

7. If there were abortions, stillbirths, or children who died postnatally, what were the reasons if known?

8. What illnesses involving other children or relatives, especially in the area of neurologic dysfunction, are present or have occurred in the past?

9. Have there been, or are there, learning problems or behavioral disturbances in other family members?

GESTATIONAL AND PERINATAL HISTORY

1. What problems were encountered in pregnancy?

2. What medications were taken during pregnancy?

3. What type of delivery was used, and who delivered the child?

4. Were there complications encountered during the delivery?

5. What was the baby's birth weight?

6. What was the baby's condition at birth. What was the Apgar score?

7. What problems did the mother experience at delivery or just afterwards?

8. What problems did the baby have after birth?

DEVELOPMENTAL HISTORY*

1. When did the baby turn over?

2. When did the baby sit alone if placed in this position?

3. When did the baby get to a sitting position unaided?

*Several instruments described later in this book offer a more detailed approach to the attainment of a developmental history.

DEVELOPMENTAL HISTORY *(cont'd)*

4. When did the baby crawl?

5. When did the child stand?

6. When did the child walk?

7. Did he walk on his toes to a conspicuous degree, and does he still do this?

8. What other gait problems have been present?

9. When did he feed himself with his fingers? with utensils? with a cup?

10. When did he learn to undress himself, put on outer garments, manage buttons, zippers and laces?

11. When was he toilet trained? Bladder and bowel? Day and night?

12. What difficulties were encountered in these areas of training?

13. When did he use single words, phrases, and sentences?

14. How clear or well formed was speech, and how is it presently utilized?

PAST MEDICAL HISTORY

1. What feeding problems were encountered in the past?

2. Did the baby have colic?

3. Have there been any significant injuries, illnesses, or operations?

4. How did the child sleep, and what sleep problems are now evident?

5. Have parents reported problems with child's hearing?

6. Has anyone else questioned the patient's hearing ability?

7. Has there been any otologic illness?

8. What eye problems has the child had?

9. Has the patient used glasses? Has there been any strabismus? Has there been any eye therapy?

10. Has the patient experienced any seizure with or without fever?

11. Have there been any trancelike episodes or minor lapses which could be petit mal or other seizure fragments?

12. Has the patient shown any unusual reaction to medications?

13. What neurologic complaints are present? such as headache, vomiting, poor balance, double vision, dizziness, weakness, numbness.

PSYCHOSOCIAL HISTORY

1. What difficulties have the parents had in managing the child now and in the past?

2. What problems does the child evidence with his siblings now and in the past?

3. What problems does the child have in relating to and playing with other children now and in the past?

4. What sleeping problems are encountered?

5. What feeding problems are noted?

6. Does the child demonstrate temper tantrums?

7. What does the child enjoy doing the most?

8. What makes the child angry?

9. What is the capability of the child in varied play activities involving gross motor control?

10. What is the capability of the child in play activities requiring fine motor control?

11. Is attention span short?

12. Does the child seem unduly impulsive?

13. Does the child lack self-control?

14. Is the child overly active?

15. Does the child react out-of-proportion when faced with problems?

EDUCATIONAL HISTORY

1. Did the child go to nursery school?

2. What problems were encountered in nursery school?

3. What kindergarten did the child attend?

4. What problems were noted in kindergarten?

5. Where is the child presently placed in school?

6. Has he been retained?

7. How does he behave in class?

8. What is his reading level?

EDUCATIONAL HISTORY *(cont'd)*

9. What are his arithmetic skills?

10. Does he have difficulty with handwriting?

11. Does he have difficulty in getting along with his classmates?

12. Has he seen the school psychologist or other special educational personnel?

13. Has he received special help at school?

14. What do his report cards reveal?

15. How does the child react to going to school now and in the past?

REACREATIONAL ADJUSTMENT

1. How does the child play with his peers?

2. Does he prefer to play with younger children?

3. Does he fight frequently with his playmates?

4. Did he have difficulty in learning to ride a bicycle?

5. Did he have difficulty in learning to skip?

6. Did he have problems in learning to throw or catch?

7. Does he show uncertainty in hand usage in throwing or kicking?

8. Does he become easily overstimulated in play?

9. Does he seem to be overly energetic or overly exuberant in his play activities?

10. Are there complaints from other mothers in the neighborhood in relation to play with their children or play in or near their homes?

FRAGMENTING INSTRUMENTATION
(NORMATIVE AND NON-NORMATIVE)

Many multi-handicapped youngsters are difficult, if not impossible, to assess using traditional normative devices. Instruments such as the Stanford Binet and Wechsler Intelligence Test (revised), have been normed on a population quite different from that represented by youngsters in a multi-handicapped class. Traditional instrumentation places emphasis on verbal and motor responses, the very areas in which the multi-handicapped child is often weakest. Many evaluators do, however, use parts of normative instruments to gain specific information which is then used to help paint a clearer picture of the child. The very real problem faced today by evaluators having to assess and make recommendations for a program for the multi-handicapped child results from their having been trained in the use of standardized or normative assessment devices, including traditional intellectual and academic or performance based. They have used normative tests, incorporated them into their assessment procedures, and are apt to be unfamiliar with methods and materials related to informal assessment.

In assessing various domains of the multi-handicapped, we come to the issue of the accuracy of such things as developmental age, mental age, and IQ. Psychologists are most often the individuals accused of unfairly using tests with children who have sensory and/or response limitations. Often, children are given inappropriate tests because of their handicap with consequent invalidity resulting. Guidelines will follow for arriving at ways to provide a more functionally descriptive assessment of the child while still taking into account concepts such as developmental age and mental age. The most obvious way to deal with a child having a particular handicap is to select a test or a portion of a test that should result in a relatively unbiased assessment of his developmental levels in as many domains as possible. Examples of unbiased assessment include (1) giving hearing-impaired children a nonverbal test such as the Leiter International Performance Scale, the Hiskey Nebraska Test of Learning Aptitude, or the Wechsler Performance Scale; or (2) giving a blind child the verbal portion of the Wechsler tests. By contrast, many nonverbal or speech-impaired youngsters have been given Stanford-Binet intelligence tests which draw heavily upon verbal skills thus rendering a measure of the cognitive domain invalid. Many professionals have moved away from giving one complete "test" to multi-handicapped youngsters, opting instead to "fragment" their assessment, using parts of several instruments to help portray a complete picture of the child. If, as a result of one's observations, it becomes apparent that the child's sensory and/or response limitations prevent the administration of a given test with conventional administration and scoring, then the following ideas may prove to be helpful.

The examiner(s) may want to modify the test item(s) in order that the child can indicate that he is capable of responding correctly but simply cannot do so in the prescribed manner. Such modifications in administration might include enabling the child to point, allowing extra time, or taking into account motor dysrhythmia in assessing fine and gross motor levels. In some cases, when assessing the cognitive domain, the examiner may want to administer an item in a multiple choice manner with the child giving some indication of when the correct answer has been given. Such indication may be given through a yes or no response, an eye blink, finger wiggle, or whatever response is within the child's capability. There has been a successful attempt to modify the items on the Stanford-Binet Scale from years two through four so that all of them can be administered using either a yes-no or pointing response (Sattler 1973). IN ALL CASES, MODIFICATIONS IN ADMINISTRATION SHOULD BE REPORTED.

The selective administration and modification techniques can be used with a variety of instruments. When the evaluator has done as much testing as is needed or possible, the data should be organized in a developmental order in an effort to gain a fairly accurate understanding of where the child is across all domains along the developmental continuum.

The examiner should look at the child's successes up to the point where his first failure occurred; if the data is organized in an approximately developmental order, then the point just below the level at which the first failure occurs constitutes a basal level estimate. At this point, there may be a need to use clinical judgment by determining whether or not failures beyond the point resulted from particular sensory and/or response limitation. If so, the developmental level of that domain could be reported as a range rather than a specific age, e.g. 3-5 to 4-2. This range would allow for projected successes clearly based upon the judgment of the examiner(s).

It should be re-emphasized that this more flexible method of using assessment tools requires *justification* based on specific observations of sensory and/or response limitations. The examiner must show cause as to why there was a deviation from standard procedure.

THE FAMILY AS AN INFORMATION SOURCE

One of the numerous ways in which assessment of multi-handicapped youngsters differs from that of less severe youngsters is in the assessment of family dynamics as they relate to the handicapped child. Teachers stressed the importance of the assessor, whether he/she be a psychologist, supervisor, or teacher, becoming familiar with the dynamics of the family. The person conducting the assessment should get into the home and interview *both* parents in that setting. One teacher interviewed during the course of our research suggested "that a multiply-handicapped child can be a disaster to a family." This statement lends validity to the concept of assessing the family dynamics as they revolve around the child. Both formal and informal approaches are recommended for home/parent interviews. Structured parent interview forms such as the "Outline for Parent Interview" seen later in this chapter provide a constancy factor allowing the person conducting the parent interview to be certain of gaining specific information. This type of interview form combined with the skill of the interviewer allows for the possibility of gaining much incidental information as the interviewee(s) elaborate beyond the bounds of specific questions presented to them. The combination of formal and informal assessment in the home provides a dimension which, if absent, could radically change the educational and rehabilitative program for the child in the classroom.

BEING AWARE OF PARENTAL "MIND SETS"

Persons working with parents of handicapped children have undoubtedly realized the pay off in being aware of and understanding "mind sets" of parents of handicapped children. This is a major consideration in the assessment process which is tied directly to interviewing, one of the integral parts of assessment. Awareness on the part of the interviewer of possible stages through which parents evolve in adjusting to their child's handicap can greatly facilitate the interviewing process and are offered to the reader for that purpose. Interviewers moving into the session without an awareness of possible parent mind sets stand to gain less from the interview than one who has stopped to consider "where the parent(s) are coming from."

Responses and behaviors of parents of handicapped children are predicted on the concept of grief related to a loss, the loss of the parents' opportunity to live vicariously through the accomplishments of their children. Parents tend to develop expectations for their children, to develop fantasies around these expectations, and the handicapping condition often serves to shatter these dreams causing a feeling of grief often in proportion to the importance of the expectations developed by the parents. A sequence of parental mind sets, not necessarily in the following order and not always including each of the affective states to be mentioned, often occurs.

1. FAILURE TO BELIEVE. Parents won't accept a diagnosis and will continue to shop for a new diagnosis or cure. Parents may also minimize the seriousness of the handicap as they develop coping mechanisms allowing them to deal with it.
2. SELF-BLAME. An overwhelming guilt is frequently initiated by the parent. Mother — "If it had not been for something I did during the gestation period this wouldn't have happened." Father — "Something genetically incorrect must exist within me."
3. ANGER AND SELF-PITY. These two emotions are often closely aligned. Parents feel helpless and unable to change the handicapping condition. This helplessness often develops into either anger or pity. Parents will displace their anger onto the professional, the spouse, or the institution. Persons conducting the interview should be prepared for this and should be ready to deal with it. Self-pity and/or depression can be expected from parents of handicapped children and should be permitted as the parents wrestle with how to cope with their problem. Interviewers should note these parental characteristics since they may be used later in setting up parent groups once your teaching pro-

gram is underway.

4. GIVING AND SHARING. A common type of parental reaction which usually takes place following failure to believe, self blame, and anger and self pity, is seen as the parent volunteers to help other parents of handicapped or as they begin to help teachers and other educational personnel. They may also become very involved with their handicapped child's activities or they may offer their child for research purposes.

With an understanding of the existing parental states of mind, the interviewer should be able to procede more efficiently with the interview being able to anticipate possible emotions or behaviors generated as a result of the perceptions. Now the interviewer is ready to gain information from the parents which will allow for a better understanding of the child and will lead consequently to a more meaningful educational program. To help the interviewer gain specific information regarding the child, a specific format should be used that will insure thoroughness in gaining information. The outline listed is offered to the reader as an example of types of interview questions to be asked and will add considerably to the material gained from the assessment.

OUTLINE FOR PARENT INTERVIEW

Inform the parent that you are going to ask some very specific questions about the child's day:

1. On a school day, how does your child awaken? (May need to give suggestions, i.e. Does the child awaken by himself?)
2. How does your child prepare himself for the day? (i.e. Who selects the clothing?)
3. Does the child get ready quickly or does the child require continual reminding?
4. Does the child eat breakfast? Who prepares breakfast? Any hassles at this time?
5. Does the child watch the time and leave promptly or do you have to remind him frequently? Has your child ever

refused to go to school?
6. Does your child come home for lunch? (Repeat questions 4 and 5 if the child has lunch at home.)
7. What happens after school?, i.e. What does the child do first? Next?
8. What occurs at dinner time?
   a. Does the family eat together?
   b. Is the child on time?
   c. Any problems during dinner?
   d. Does he/she participate in family conversation during meals?
9. What happens after dinner?
10. What happens at bedtime? Does he/she get ready for bed and go to bed when requested?
11. What does the child do on weekends? (May need to break the weekend into specific days and period of time.)
12. Does the family have a chance to do many things together? (May need to suggest examples, i.e. shopping, movies.)
13. Does your child spend time with friends?
    a. How much time?
    b. How many friends?
    c. How do you feel about your child's friends?
14. Does your child belong to any groups or organizations? i.e. Scouts, Y, after school activities, sports.
15. Does your child have any particular interests or hobbies?
16. Does your child get an allowance?
    a. Is the allowance earned, or does he ever earn money?
    b. How does the child manage the money?
17. Does your child have specific chores?
    a. What?
    b. How often?
    c. Any hassles about chores? How does your child avoid chores? i.e. refuses, argues, disappears.
18. How do you generally discipline your child?
    a. How often?
    b. Does it work?
19. If you could change one thing about your child, what would it be?

20. What does your child do well?
21. What do you like about your child?

With the conclusion of the parent interview you now have information about the child's past and present behavior which can be combined with other formal and informal assessment material to provide a comprehensive understanding of the child.

ASSESSMENT RELATED TO PARENT GROUPS

Another aspect of assessment which should be considered according to teachers working with the multi-handicapped is the responsibility to assess parent needs for the purpose of possibly providing ongoing parent groups. Parents of multi-handicapped children are often quite heterogeneous in terms of personal needs and may have as their only homogenous factor the possession of a multi-handicapped child. A major part, then, of an assessment program should be a parental needs assessment to be used in the development of group meetings for the parents. Perhaps the best way to develop an understanding of parent needs is simply to ask them what they would like to discuss with other parents in a group setting. While the topics can be expected to be diverse, the good which is inherent in well-run groups is typically reported to be increased information and understanding of the parents' handicapped child and a "good feeling" after sharing information with other parents experiencing the same or similar problems.

ASSESSMENT OF TEACHER-STAFF NEEDS

An important aspect of assessment that might not be considered within the realm of assessment by some is the determination of the emotional and support needs of the teachers and aids of the multi-handicapped child. Information gained from teachers and aids suggested that they often felt isolated from other faculty and felt either unprepared or unsupported in terms of handling many of the serious parent/child/family problems indigenous to the multi-handicapped population. Persons involved in establishing an assessment program and consequently an educational program for multi-handicapped children should pay particular attention to the pre-service and in-service educational needs of teachers and aides and, in particular, should make ongoing provision for support type meetings which will do at least two major things: (1) they will allow teachers/aides to get direct, technical advice on problems related to their class; and (2) they will allow for plain, old catharsis, giving the teacher an opportunity to share her feelings and concerns.

CONCLUSION

Legislation has very directly affected methods of assessment in special education. The emphasis which has been given to providing a free and appropriate education for all school-aged youngsters has created a need to move toward functional, descriptive, non-normative assessment and away from normative assessment describing children in terms of "scores." This chapter has attempted to provide considerations and guidelines to persons interested in developing an assessment program for multi-handicapped youngsters. Viewing the multi-handicapped child as one who is very individualistic in terms of needs, assessment approaches should be developed to fully provide an understanding of the multi-handicapped child's strengths and weaknesses in a variety of areas. Ongoing diagnosis as opposed to a single diagnostic session provides a more comprehensive picture of the child. The ongoing assessment should be multi-disciplinary in nature drawing from the expertise of more than one specialist. Combining normative and non-normative data and supplementing this data with assessment information provided by a physician, information gained through parent interviews, and data obtained through the use of such formal items as medical developmental histories and screening checklists helps educators design meaningful, prescriptive programs for youngsters.

Finally, assessment models need to be developed that are functional in nature (describing children's adaptable behavior in a wide variety of domains or describing him as he relates to his present world) while attempting to suggest the next considerations in the remedial hierarchy.

PART II — GUIDELINES FOR ASSESSMENT
OF MULTI-HANDICAPPED CHILDREN

A good assessment program for multi-handicapped young-sters must have clearly stated objectives which fall within a sound, organizational framework for assessment. To this point in the text, the reader has been made aware of numerous con-siderations and concepts related to the multi-handicapped child, the assessment of that child, and the milieu in which he interacts. This information is necessary before assuming the task of assembling an assessment program for the multi-handicapped youngster. The designer of the assessment pro-gram must be aware of the many contiguous points associated with this type of child before he/she begins the task of de-signing the assessment program. With a major part of the "ges-talt" in mind, including awareness of such things as evolving legislation, realizing the value of ongoing diagnosis, involving parents, recognizing the limitations of normative assessment instrumentations, and being able to assess parent and teacher needs, the educator should then be able to establish his purpose and objectives for a multi-factored evaluation. Purpose, unlike that for nonhandicapped, could include a *training*-related phi-losophy as well as the more typical academic orientation so that the purpose of an assessment program for the multi-handicapped might be stated in this manner. Individualized assessment across all domains should be conducted for the pur-pose of determining strengths and weaknesses which should be remediated through training and through academic pursuits with the ultimate goal being one of making the child more adaptive to his environment. The following objectives of the assessment program might be considered by persons involved in establishing an assessment program for the multi-handicapped (Matey 1975):

1. To collect data from a variety of sources, e.g. medical and school records, standardized tests, criterion references tests, interviews, and observation.
2. To collect data which identifies specific academic and

social skill strengths and weaknesses.

3. To collect data which establishes the child's present levels of performance in a variety of areas, e.g., academic, social, personal and emotional functioning, cognitive functioning, motor skills, communication skills, and adaptive behavior.

4. To collect data which identifies vocational and occupational needs of the child.

5. To collect medical information from all available sources which can be used to determine if further medical evaluation and/or intervention should be discussed with medical professionals.

6. To collect educationally relevant and descriptive data which will assure that the assessed child is not unnecessarily labeled as handicapped.

7. To collect educationally relevant and descriptive data which can be used for determining the child's individualized educational plan and for developing initial short-term instructional objectives.

8. To formulate a written report which shall contain a summary of the reason for the evaluation, assessment procedures and findings, description of any factors that may have adversely affected the child's performance, present levels of functioning, and specific recommendations for the child's educational program.

To insure completeness in functional assessment and to attain the aforementioned goals of assessment, persons developing and maintaining functional assessment programs should consider the following diagnostic plan which depicts the major components necessary for complete functional assessment.

FUNCTIONAL ASSESSMENT MODEL

Screening

Utilization of a screening checklist will allow the assessor to observe a number of behavioral components of the child making possible the development of an overall initial diagnostic impression and aiding in defining the problem. A sample observational checklist is included later in this chapter.

Knowledge of Developmental Levels

Utilization of developmental levels allows for the understanding of the child along two continua, one using the child as his own frame of reference, the second comparing the child to a mean level relative to his chronological peers. In discussing maturation and learning, Piaget (1964) comments on cultural factors (learning experiences) which delay or accelerate development: "Maturation doesn't explain everything, because the average ages at which these stages appear (the average chronological ages) vary a great deal from one society to another (Medvedeff 1969). A major point, however, is that these stages are invariant in terms of ordering, regardless of cultural factors.

With maturation and learning processes being complexly interrelated, it is important for those persons conducting multi-factored assessments to have a means by which developmental levels in the major domains can be determined. There have been for years a number of developmental schedules available which describe "normal" or "average" behavior per month or year of life. In addition to developmental schedules, assessment devices exist that allow examiners to look at behaviors and responses in various domains for the purpose of determining an age level. The following material is mentioned below to provide for the reader a reference to various materials related to the concept of developmental assessment and includes related readings as well as specific developmental schedules and instruments that yield developmental ages.

Developmental History

A good developmental history should include information about the family, gestational and perinatal history, developmental history, medical history, psychosocial history, educational history, and a section on the child's recreational activities.

Cumulative Data

Often multi-handicapped children have been assessed previously by other professionals. Much time can be saved and much information gained by taking advantage of existing cumulative records on the child.

Goals and Objectives of Parents

If parents are not in accord with goals and objectives stemming from the diagnostic findings of the assessor, remedial programming becomes difficult, if not impossible. In defining the problem, parent input is vital. Chapter Nine discusses the legal aspects of parental involvement.

Development of Diagnostic Plan

Once the aforementioned steps in defining the problem have been covered, a determination can be made regarding the assessment plan. Instrumentation can be selected, and specific domains and processes can be isolated for more careful assessment and study. Defining the problem is vital in providing direction for the remainder of the functional assessment and is necessary to help determine which of the following factors to invest in as the assessment is planned and implemented:

Medical	Fine Motor
Vision	Personal/Social
Auditory	Cognitive
Language	Achievement and/or Academic
Gross Motor	Vocational

MAKING PLACEMENT AND PROGRAMMING DECISIONS

Information related to these domains will have been gathered through the use of such resources as physicians, medical/developmental history, observation, screening checklists, parent interview, normative and non-normative assessment (or a fragmentation of each) and now must be pulled together in a meaningful way to help the child. The process of interpreting the data can be facilitated by constructing a developmental profile reflecting the results of the assessment with at least two conclusions being drawn from each area assessed; the evaluator should be able to estimate *an approximate developmental level* for each domain assessed, and he should be able to *specify the skills* that seem to be indicated as representing the *next step* in the developmental sequence. The approximate developmental level should be indicated in terms of an age range with the skills specified being thought of as representing beginning educational or training goals (Matey 1975). It should be understood that the profile constructed in this manner may be somewhat tentative but will reflect collective impressions obtained in a variety of ways from various persons (at least parents and an evaluator). The profile could take the form as shown in Figure 1 (page 67), which illustrates how a developmental record of progress in domains over the years can be recorded.

The profile provides important historical documentation for future use allowing for measurement of progress over time. The chart allows for comparison of the child to himself over time or, with the use of the dotted line illustrating normal growth expectancy, the child may be compared to the other children his own age across particular domains. It may also be examined in order that a decision can be made as to which educational program in the community could best meet the child's needs. For example, a child with a severe deficit in communication skills but with near age-level skills in the other domains might be appropriately placed in a special class for children with language problems or he may be provided with special speech and language therapy. The evaluation might also reveal a child whose understanding of language is good but who cannot speak in more than one-word sentences; such information would suggest that teaching designed to permit other than verbal response modes should be used in addition to the obvious attempts to help the child learn to speak. On the other hand, a child with a severe communication handicap could also be significantly below age expectancy level in the other areas assessed. In a case such as this, it might be concluded that the child is retarded or behind in all areas assessed and might be more appropriately involved in a program for such children.

Once a placement recommendation has been made accompanied by suggestions for initial teaching goals and strategies, follow-up conferences with the child's parents and school personnel can facilitate transition into the program. Ultimately, the child's performance in an instructional setting will reveal the appropriateness of the evaluator(s)'s recommendations. However, an initial placement based on a multi-factored evaluation using the various perspectives for gathering information will result in fewer misplacements and rough beginnings for children.

The use of a developmental profile such as this illustrating assessments at ages two years and four years does at least three major things: (1) it allows educators to know where the child is developmentally across all domains; (2) it permits more meaningful remedial planning for the child within each of these domains; and (3) it provides a developmental baseline from which future improvement and regression can be measured. As an example, the chart (as displayed in Table 2-II) shows virtually no gain developmentally over a period of two years.

CONCLUSION

An assessment model stressing the importance of providing information related to a child's trainability and his adaptive behavior across all domains should be developed by persons assessing multi-handicapped youngsters. Screening checklists allow the assessor(s) to quickly pick up a picture of the child's strengths and weaknesses. Formal and informal assessment provide objective and subjective information related to the child's capability in certain domains while utilization of developmental histories, cumulative records, and input from parents, teachers, and others helps to complete the picture of the child. Construction of a profile of the child's strengths and weaknesses will add clarity to the "picture" of the child by (1) allowing for the comparison of the child to others, (2) by providing for comparison of the child to himself across several domains, and (3) by suggesting the next remedial thrust based upon existing developmental levels.

Table 2-II

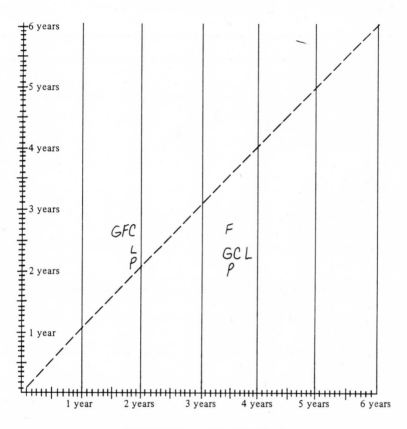

Chronological Age (Years/Months)

- - Normal Growth Expectancy
L = Language
P = Personal Social
C = Cognitive
A = Academic Achievement
F = Fine Motor
G = Gross Motor

Multiple Domain Screening Checklist

Child's Name_____ Informant_____

Age_____ Telephone Number_____

Home Address_____ Grade _____

_____ Date _____

Directions: Check in the *yes* column if there appears to be a problem in the specified behavior and check *no* if a problem does not seem to exist.

VISUAL	YES	NO
1. Eyes squint		
2. Eyes blink		
3. Eyes tic		
4. Eyes water		
5. Eye lids frequently encrusted		
6. Eyes often reddened		
7. Eyes have frequent styes		
8. Child tilts head when reading or doing paper work		
9. Child reports dizziness frequently		
10. Child reports headaches frequently		

11. Other pertinent or relative characteristics include the following:

_____

AUDITORY	YES	NO
1. Child speaks in a monotone		
2. Frequent earaches reported		
3. Words are often misarticulated		
4. Responses inappropriate to verbal stimulation		
5. Child asks to have words, phrases, or sentences repeated		
6. Child seems to strain to hear, positioning head abnormally when others are talking		
7. Child accents wrong syllables		
8. Oral reading includes many mispronunciations		
9. Animation and reaction is often inappropriate to verbal stimulation		

10. Other pertinent or relative characteristics include the following:

_____

SPEECH

	YES	NO
1. Child stammers or stutters		
2. Child makes sound substitutions (*w* for *r*, *t* for *d*)		
3. Speech contains "baby talk"		
4. Child has tendency to lisp		
5. Child does not use consonant and vowel sounds in all positions in one- or two-syllable words		
6. Child does not use consonant and vowel sounds in all positions in three- or four-syllable words		
7. Child does not use all consonant and vowel sounds in phrases and sentences		

8. Other pertinent or relative characteristics include the following:

LANGUAGE

	YES	NO
1. Child unable to gesture meaningfully to simple verbal requests		
2. Child unable to follow verbal directions which are supplemented with gestures		
3. Child unable to follow single verbal directions without gestures		
4. Child unable to respond with simple words or phrases to questions concerning concepts (e.g. Do you like candy?)		
5. Child unable to answer specific questions based on verbalized material (e.g. What did I just say?)		
6. Child unable to carry on a conversation		

7. Other pertinent or relative behaviors include the following:

LISTENING

	YES	NO
1. Child responds to questions and comments incorrectly or inappropriately		
2. Child unable to perform actions or tasks in response to individually given instructions		
3. Child unable to follow directions when given to a group		
4. Child unable to correctly respond to questions covering material spoken less than one minute before		
5. Child unable to correctly respond to questions concerning material spoken more than one minute before		
6. Child unable to carry out two or less directions (e.g. Open the door and bring me the box on the table)		

7. Child unable to carry out three-step directions
8. Child unable to carry out four-step directions
9. Child is incapable of paraphrasing
10. Other pertinent or relative behaviors include the following:

BEHAVIORAL FACTORS   YES   NO

1. Child seems to blank-out at times
2. Child shows frequent perseverative behavior in speech
3. Child shows frequent perseverative behavior in motion
4. Child engages in ritualistic behavior
5. Child stares a lot
6. Child wanders aimlessly without purpose
7. Child has difficulty understanding what is said
8. Child has difficulty in expressing self
9. The quantity and quality of the child's work varies greatly
10. Child tends to forget what seemingly has been learned
11. Child has difficulty with rote memory
12. Child has difficulty with problem solving
13. Child seems to shake and shiver at times
14. Other pertinent or relative behaviors include the following:

PSYCHO-MOTOR   YES   NO

1. Child appears hypoactive (slow and listless in all settings)
2. Child appears impulsive (lacks reflectivity)
3. Child has poor attention span
4. Child has difficulty hopping, running, jumping
5. Child has difficulty coloring, pasting, printing, drawing
6. Child is clumsy and/or awkward
7. Child shows perseverative motor behavior (head banging, rocking, fingering, hitting self)
8. Child is hyperactive (constantly in motion in all settings)
9. Child's musculature is hypotonic (flaccid)
10. Child's musculature is hypertonic (tense or rigid)
11. Child's movements are spastic in nature
12. Child's movements are labored (athetoid)
13. Child exhibits lack of balance in performing normal motor tasks
14. Tremulousness is evident in motor behavior
15. Other pertinent or relative behaviors include the following:

SOCIAL-EMOTIONAL FACTORS

	YES	NO
1. Child displays a proneness to emotional outbursts		
2. Child shows major mood swings (ecstasy to depression)		
3. Child soils self		
4. Child wets self		
5. Child demonstrates abnormal fear		
6. Child seems to tune-out surroundings for marked periods of time		
7. Child is destructive		
8. Child displays verbal aggressivity to peers		
9. Child displays physical aggressivity to peers		
10. Child has poor relations with peers		
11. Child has poor relations with adults		
12. Child appears emotionally "flat" (no emotional peaks or valleys)		
13. Child sleeps in class		
14. Child constantly complains of physical ailments		
15. Child engages in high-anxiety behaviors (nail biting, excessive talking)		
16. Child needs structure and guidance		
17. Child lacks self-initiative (waits to be told)		
18. Child quits easily		
19. Child cries easily		
20. Child exaggerates to excess		
21. School attendance poor		
22. Child lies frequently		
23. Child used profanity excessively		
24. Child exhibits feelings of insecurity		
25. Child prefers to be left alone and withdraws from others		
26. Child exhibits little self-confidence		
27. Child exhibits inappropriate affect (e.g. laughing or crying at the wrong times)		
28. Child enjoys inflicting pain on self		
29. Child exhibits compulsive behavior (e.g. excessive hand washing)		

30. Other pertinent or relative characteristics include the following:

Appendix B

Assessment Instrumentation

Bayley Scales of Infant Development
These scales provide discriminatory assessment of mental and motor behavior from two months to the developmental age of thirty months.

Cain-Levin Social Competency Scale
Standardized on a group of mentally retarded children, this scale assesses five major areas from five to thirteen years. Self-help, initiative, social skills, communication, and a total global functioning score are derived using third-party information gained from the primary care giver.

Comprehensive Developmental Evaluation Chart
This chart provides for assessment of developmental ages from birth to three years in eleven areas: reflexes, gross motor, manipulation, vision, feeding, receptive language, expressive language, cognitive/social, muscle tone, hips, hearing.

Cattell Infant Intelligence Scale
The Cattell allows for the measurement of developmental age from three months to thirty months providing a developmental age but no specific age related to domains.

Developmental Activities Screening Inventory
This is a teacher administered screening instrument which is designed to yield developmental levels from six months to sixty months in the areas of general cognitive adaptive functioning levels.

Developmental Profile
The Developmental Profile is an inventory of skills which has been designed to assess a child's development from birth to pre-adolescence. The inventory depicts a child's developmental age level in the following five areas: physical age, self-help age, social age, academic age, communication age.

Learning Accomplishment Profile LAP
The LAP provides developmental ages from one month through six years in the domains of gross motor, fine motor, language, cognition, social, and self-help skills.

Maxfield Buchholz Scale for the Blind
This social development scale, birth through six years, is an adaptation of Vineland Social Maturity Scale and evaluates social development in the areas of general motor development, dressing, eating, locomotion, socialization, communication, and occupation.

Merrill-Palmer Scales of Mental Development
These scales assess not only the child's cognitive abilities but also expressive and receptive language and fine and gross motor skills. The age range runs from two to six years.

Minnesota Child Development Inventory

This inventory utilizes the mother's observations of her child's development in arriving at developmental ages from six months to six and one-half years in the areas of general development, gross motor, fine motor, expressive language, comprehension-conceptual, situation comprehension, self-help, personal-social.

Ordinal Scales of Psychological Development

These scales measure cognitive development and has a series of six ordinal scales based on Piagetian observations of sensory-motor schemes birth to twenty-four months. Six scales include visual pursuit and the permanence of objects, the development of means for obtaining desired environmental events, development of vocal and gestural unitation, development of schemes for relating to objects, development of operational causality, and the construction of object relations in space.

Tests for Auditory Comprehension

This language development test measures auditory comprehension and permits assignment of children to developmental levels three to seven years. Performance of items requires only a pointing response and scales assess morphology, semantics, and syntax.

Vineland Social Maturity Scale

The Vineland allows for a broad measure of a person's capabilities and ranges from birth through adulthood. It assesses a person's general skills in self-help, occupation, self-management, social maturity, and communication.

SUGGESTED READINGS

Gesell, A. *The First Five Years of Life: A Guide to the Study of the Preschool Child.* New York, Harper, 1940.
  This book, although dated, contains age-wise descriptions of the first five years of life.
Gesell, A., and Ilg, F. L. *The Child From Five to Ten.* New York, Harper, 1946.
  Included in this book are descriptions of physical growth and mental growth focusing on years five to ten.
Ilg, F., and Ames, L. B. Child Behavior from Birth to Ten. New York, Har-Row.
  This book discusses behavioral characteristics pertinent to growth stages through the first ten years.
Medvedeff, E., and Dearth, B. *New Dimensions in Learning.* Akron, Ohio, Prescriptive Educational Systems, 1974.
  Chapter Seven of this book discusses the topic of growth trends and provides sequences of behavior from 0 to 9 years across the domains of

motor communication-listening, and personal-social.

White, B. *The First Three Years of Life.* Englewood Cliffs, New Jersey, P-H, 1975.

This book looks at details of development during the first three years of life. While not attempting to discuss specific expected behaviors at given points of time. Much excellent material is included related to the education of children during the first three years.

REFERENCES

Alpern, Gerald D., and Boll, Thomas J. *A Manual for the Developmental Profile.* Aspen, Colorado, Psychological Development Publications, 1972.

Bayley, Nancy. *Manual for Bayley Scales of Infant Development.* New York, Psych Corp, 1969.

Cain, Leo; Levine, Samuel; and Freeman, Elzey. *A Manual for the Cain-Levine Social Competency Scale.* Palo Alto, California, Consulting Psychol, 1977.

Carrow, Elizabeth. *A Manual for the Tests for Auditory Comprehension of Language.* Austin, Texas, Learning Concepts, 1973.

Cattell, Psyche. *A Manual for Cattell Infant Intelligence Scale.* Dallas, The Psychological Corporation, 1960.

Ciba Pharmaceutical Company. *Medical/Developmental History.* Summit, New Jersey, 1975.

Cliff, Shirley, et al. *Manual for Comprehensive Developmental Evaluation Chart.* El Paso, El Paso Rehabilitation Center, 1975.

Doll, E. *A Manual for the Vineland Scale of Social Maturity.* Circle Pines, Minnesota, Am Guidance, 1969.

Dubose, Rebecca F., and Langley, Mary Beth. *Developmental Activities Screening Inventory.* Boston, Teaching Resources Corporation, 1977.

Elkind, David. *A Sympathetic Understanding of the Child: Birth to Sixteen.* Boston, Allyn, 1971.

Gesell, A., and Ilg, F. L. *The Child From Five to Ten.* New York, Harper, 1946.

Gesell, A. *The First Five Years of Life.* New York, Harper, 1940.

Hiskey, Marshall S. *Manual for the Hiskey-Nebraska Test of Learning Aptitude.* Lincoln, Nebraska, Union College Press, 1966.

Ilg, F., and Ames, L. B. *Child Behavior from Birth to Ten.* New York, Har-Row, 1955.

Ireton, Harold, and Thwing, Edward. *A Manual for the Minnesota Child Development Inventory.* Behavior Science Systems, Inc., 1972.

Kent, Louise. *Language Acquisition Program for the Retarded or Multiply Impaired.* Champaign, Illinois, Res Press, 1974.

Matey, Christopher. Guidelines for Assessment of Low Incidence Handicapped and Multi-Impaired Children. The Miami Valley

Regional Center for Handicapped Children, Dayton, Ohio, 1975.

Maxfield, K. E., and Buchholz, S. *A Social Maturity Scale for the Blind.* New York, Am Foun Blind, 1957.

Medvedeff, Eugene, and Dearth, Beverly. *New Dimensions in Learning.* Akron, Ohio, Prescriptive Educational Systems, 1969.

Merrill, Maud A., and Terman, Lewis M. *The Manual for the Stanford-Binet.* Boston, HM, 1962.

Murray, Joseph N., and New, Frank. A goal of full service for handicapped students, *Education, 98(March)*: 325-333, 1978.

Murray, Joseph N., and Wright, Elizabeth A. Consideration in establishing and maintaining severe/multiple units. *Education and Training of the Mentally Retarded, 14(February)*: 59-66, 1979.

Piaget Rediscovered. A report of the conference on cognitive studies and curriculum development. New York, Cornell University, 1964.

Positive Education Program. *Parent Questionnaire.* Cleveland, Ohio, 1975.

Program Standards for Special Education, effective June 30, 1973, and Standards for Due Process and Procedural Safeguards for Handicapped Children and Youth, effective August 28, 1976. Ohio Department of Education, Columbus, Ohio.

Sanford, Anne R. *A Manual for the Learning Accomplishment Profile.* Winston-Salem, Kaplan School Supply Corp., 1974.

Sattler, Jerome M. *Assessment of Children's Intelligence.* Philadelphia, Saunders, 1974.

Stutsman, Rachel. *Guide for Administering the Merrill-Palmer Scale of Mental Tests.* Los Angeles, Western Psych, 1948.

U.S. Congress. House. Education of the Handicapped Amendments of 1974. Education Amendments of 1974, Sections 611-621, Public Law 93-380 (HR 69), 93rd Congress, 2nd Session, 1974.

U.S. Congress. Senate. Education for All Handicapped Children Act of 1975. Public Law 94-142 (S.6), 94th Congress, 1st Session, 1975.

Uzgiris, I.C., and Hunt, J.M. *A Manual for Assessment in Infancy: Ordinal Scales of Psychological Development.* Urbana, Illinois, U of Ill Pr, 1975.

Wechsler, David. *Manual for the Wechsler Intelligence Scale for Children.* New York, Psych Corp, 1949.

White, Burton L. *The First Three Years of Life.* Englewood Cliffs, New Jersey, P-H, 1975.

CHAPTER THREE

LANGUAGE ASSESSMENT — INTERVENTION WITH SPECIAL CHILDREN

GLADYS KNOTT, PH.D.

SHIFTS during the past decade in theory and perspectives on normal children's language acquisition and development necessitate examination and modification in traditional views and procedures for assessing and ameliorating children's problems in communication. One of the shifts involves a movement away from emphasis on the child's syntactic development as a primary exemplar of communication efficiency to a focus on the child's expression of semantic intent or meaning in social interactions. Another shift in perspective on normal language acquisition and development relates to children's use of language. Within the language-in-use framework, children's utterances are not articulated merely as a result of rule learning behavior; rather, they are expressed to achieve goals in social contexts. The theoretical constructs and conceptual models underlying these perspectives preclude use of standardized tests that focus on language in isolation to determine the nature of children's communication problems. The formulations infer that such information is best obtained through direct observation and analysis of children's communicative behavior in various social interactions and contexts. In this view, phonological, semantic, syntactic, and pragmatic aspects of communicative behavior are not ends in themselves. Rather, they are parts of the whole of communicative competence and serve as contributing factors which involve the child to communicate in a variety of situations.

To facilitate understanding of new directions in identification, assessment, intervention, and evaluation of children's communication problems, the initial focus of this chapter is a summary of recent contributions to the study of child language.

From the discussion of recent contributions to our understanding of children's communicative development, the reader will discern the need to evaluate and then to formulate alternatives to traditional approaches to diagnosing and remediating children's language problems. In this respect, the second section of the chapter provides a discussion of traditional assessment procedures and their inherent problems and limitations. In the third section of the chapter, a model for representing elements of communicative behavior on which language assessment-intervention procedures can be developed is proposed. The fourth section suggests principles for developing and implementing language assessment-intervention procedures with cerebral palsied, deaf-blind, and children with autisticlike behaviors who manifest difficulties in communicative behavior. Finally, in the fifth section, the role of parents and professionals is examined with respect to language assessment-intervention.

UNDERLYING PREMISE

The reader needs to be aware of an underlying assumption that influences the content of this chapter. It relates to traditional descriptions of many exceptional children's linguistic behavior as elements which are integral to etiology of developmental problems. That is, etiological factors serve as the basis for describing linguistic behavior. It is the premise of this chapter that etiological factors surrounding cerebral palsy, deaf-blindness, and child autism influence communicative development but that etiological factors do not serve to formulate language assessment-intervention procedures. The basis for program structure is a description of the child's communicative behavior.

DISCOVERING LANGUAGE ACQUISITION
AND DEVELOPMENT

The publication of *Syntactic Structures* (Chomsky 1957) is often described as the beginning of a revolutionary period in the study of child language. It marked the collapse of stimulus-response psychology to explain initial language acquisition. For decades, psychologists had held that children's verbal activity is shaped by training, that children begin with clean cerebral slates, and that linguistic systems are built and recorded on the slates. This empiricist's view held that children learn language through cultural exposure, similar to how they learn to dance.

In contrast to the empiricist's view, Chomsky maintained that children are born with an innate capacity to learn language. Genetic endowment enables children to understand rules which govern comprehension and production of linguistic utterances. From language models in the environment, the child discovers rules by which syntactic structures are generated. Thus, linguistic rule learning enables the child to develop an efficient communication system or one comparable to models provided in the environment. The marked contrasts between stimulus-response psychology and the new "psycholinguistic" framework launched a new era in the study of child language. Phonological development (Ferguson and Garnica, 1975), syntax (Chomsky 1957, 1965), semantics (Bloom 1970, 1973; Brown 1973; Schlesinger 1971; Fillmore 1968) and pragmatics (Halliday 1973, 1975; Dore 1975) evolved as major topics in a complex effort to explain the child's development of communicative behavior.[1] Highlighting major milestones, consideration is now given to these areas.

PHONOLOGICAL DEVELOPMENT

The infant and young child's utterance of sound is a subject of curiosity and controversy. However, the correlation between pre-verbal and verbal utterances, the assumption that the absence of vocalizations during infancy may suggest language retardation and the assumption that the character of the child's early vocalizations may signal problems in intellectual and psychosocial development, are offered as justification for concern (Winitz 1969). Further justification comes from knowledge that phonological aspects of linguistic behavior, such as

[1]Other sources of extensive information include Greene (1972), Muma (1978), Foss and Hakes (1978), Ingram (1976), and Moorehead and Moorehead (1976).

pauses, juncture, stress, and intonation, are integral features of the meaning of communicative behavior. Curiosity, concern, and controversy about children's phonological development resulted in many theories of acquisition. Several are summarized.

Ferguson and Garnica (1975) examined four types of theories pertaining to the child's development of phonology. According to the authors, behaviorist theories subscribe to the role of reinforcement and accord with learning theory and psychoanalysis; structuralist theories explain phonological development in terms of linguistic universals or rules which govern structural changes in language. Natural phonology theory proposes an innate structure for the acquisition and development of the sound system of language. Finally, prosodic theory, the most recent contribution, stresses the importance of auditory perception and role of linguistic input from the environment. Ferguson and Garnica concluded that the theories are incompatible, that "they cannot all be right" (p. 174) and that factual data are needed to resolve issues and questions.

Ingram (1976) described historical contributions to phonological theory and advanced an explanation of phonological development in young children which corresponds to Piagetian stages of cognitive development. During the sensori-master period, the infant engages in pre-linguistic vocalizations. These result in the child's initial utterances, approximately the first fifty words. The period of concrete operations is characterized by an expanded repertoire of speech sounds, by misarticulation of phonological elements, and by the child's ability to represent experience through linguistic symbols. During the intuitional subperiod, the child completes the phonetic inventory and begins to use longer words. This period is followed by concrete operations when derivatives of language structure are learned and when the child acquires morphophonemic rules of verbal behavior. Finally, the child masters spelling during the period of formal operations. Ingram cautioned that the periods of development are tentative and subject to modification.

DeVilliers and deVilliers (1978) considered three approaches to the child's development of speech sounds. One approach viewed the child's production of sounds as approximations of adult speech sounds with measures of frequency and accuracy of production. The second approach considered the child's acquisition of phonemes (types of sounds) that distinguish between words and distinctive features (acoustic properties) that distinguish between different phonemes. Phonemic and distinctive feature analysis permit determination of the child's knowledge of articulatory elements generated by speakers of all languages. Characterizing the processes by which the child translates adult speech sounds to indicate consistent use of certain forms at different stages of development constitutes the third approach. Through this approach, individual differences and universals which characterize phonological processes and development in children have been found. Particularly, this approach has appeal for application with exceptional children, and the interested reader is referred to the primary source.

It is clear from the discussion that young children's phonological development is not well understood. There is no consensus as to what occurs when or how. Data-based investigations of large samples of children's phonological behavior are needed to resolve some issues. Questions that address relations between children's phonological behavior and other components of linguistic behavior remain for future research.

EARLY LINGUISTIC DEVELOPMENT

Syntax

As stated earlier, Chomsky (1957, 1965) was a forerunner in researchers' attempts to explain children's syntactical development as an active and systematic process. What Chomsky's theory of generative transformational grammar suggested is that the child is born with an innate Language Acquisition Device (LAD) which includes basic linguistic universals. Through the child's application of the universals, such as symbolizations of grammatical structures and classifications of hierarchical relations, onto language models in the environment a grammatical system is induced. Transformations, such as embedding, deletion, *wh,* and yes-no questions, are applied to basic grammatical structures to generate spoken language that approximates adult forms.

Chomsky placed primary emphasis on the child's development of syntax and, for several years following the inception of the "revolution," researchers subscribed to Chomsky's theory. Numerous descriptions of children's early utterances and development of syntax were presented as child grammars (Menyuk 1971; McNeill 1970; Carrow 1968; Lee and Canter 1971; Brown, Cazden, and Gellugi 1969). Because the major focus was devoted to explanations of grammatical relations discovered in children's linguistic behavior, semantics (or the meaning aspect of child language) was almost overlooked.

However, the perceptions and persistence of a few researchers evoked concern about "meaning" in children's linguistic utterances. Generative transformational grammar explained what children learn, that is the product; it did not explain natural language learning processes. Another criticism involved Chomsky's obvious separation of syntax and semantics. The primary emphasis on syntax did not account for systematic semantic-syntactic relationships embodied in young children's language. Still, Chomsky's theory was criticized for its inadequacy in accounting for the child's selection of appropriate items from the lexicon to generate meaningful spoken language. Chomsky's nativistic, reductionist framework attributed too much to the child's innate capacity. What was needed was a linguistic theory that incorporated cognitive functioning in the child's acquisition and development of language.

Semantics-Syntax

Researchers' efforts to explain meaning in children's early utterances constituted the first major shift in the study of child language. Generally, Bloom (1970, 1971) is credited with the most explicit effort in this direction. In a study of several children's early utterances, Bloom found that meaning of the children's utterances could be obtained by relating them to the context of their occurrence. Semantic intent was incorporated in the utterances. For example, Bloom interpreted one child's utterance of the phrase "mommy sock" on separate occasions to discover that the child conveyed different meanings on each occasion. On one occasion, "mommy sock" denoted possessor-possession; on another occasion, the utterance denoted an agent-object grammatical relationship or meaning. From this intensive study, Bloom formulated several meaning categories of children's early linguistic structures. A complete analysis and discussion of Bloom's findings are beyond the scope of this review. The reader is referred to the 1970 publication for a comprehensive discussion.

Other child language researchers who supported the search for meaning in children's early utterances included Brown (1973), Bruner (1975), Schlesinger (1971), Bowerman (1973), and Greenfield and Smith (1976). Although the objective of explaining meaning in children's linguistic structures was common to these researchers, their approaches to the problem varied. For example, Schlesinger (1971) proposed generative semantics similar to Chomsky's transformational grammar to describe semantic intent. Bowerman (1973), and Greenfield and Smith (1976) suggested the use of case grammar — a set of rules governing the semantic roles of nouns in relation to verbs. Brown (1973) presented two stages of a proposed five-stage model explaining linguistic utterances and semantic relationships. Stage I semantic relationships, as proposed by Brown, and example utterances are presented in Table 3-I.

Table 3-I

Brown's Stage I Semantic Relations

Semantic Relations	Example
1. Agent and action	John hit, Baby eat
2. Action and object	Drink milk, Eat bread
3. Agent and object	John ball, Mommy sock
4. Action and locative	Walk home, Ride car
5. Entity and locative	Daddy work, Baby chair
6. Possessor and possession	Mommy sock, John ball
7. Entity and attributive	Red car, Baby doll
8. Demonstrative and entity	This house, That coat

In addition to semantic relations presented in Table 3-I, Brown recorded others which occurred less frequently and which were not communicated by all children in their utterances. Summarizing, Brown observed that Stage I semantic relations emerged from the child's experiences and development during the sensorimotor stage, as defined by Piaget (1950). Thus, the semantic relations of Stage I are symbolic representations of experience.

Brown described Stage II as the child's acquisition of certain grammatical morphemes, such as inflections, prepositions, articles, and case markers. These forms serve to "modulate" or adjust the semantic relations of Stage I to reflect number, time, and aspect. Through Stages III, IV, and V, as hypothesized by Brown, children's utterances become progressively more complete and include embeddings, negation, interrogatives, and coordinators, which approximate adult language behavior.

In conclusion, data-based investigations challenged old frameworks and contributed new knowledge relative to meaning in children's utterances. Researchers discovered that young children convey meaning or semantic intent based on their cognitive development and experience with objects, events, and models of language in the environment. The influence of context on children's linguistic behavior suggested further that they communicate for various reasons and social purposes. This dimension was not accounted for semantic theory although a few generative semanticists (Lakoff 1972; Postal 1972) attempted to include contextual information in their semantic systems. Daunted, psychologists yielded to sociolinguists to explain functions that language serves.

Pragmatics

The desire and need to explain children's use of language constituted another shift in the study of child language. Understanding of children's semantic intent in utterances was helpful, but it was also necessary to explain why children used certain utterances as opposed to others. This approach to child language has been linked with two currently popular terms: "pragmatics" and "sociolinguistics." The terms are used interchangeably, and it may help the reader to offer brief definitions.

Bates (1976a) defined pragmatics as the study of rules for using language in context. It is "the child's ability to select a particular type of sentence and to 'fix it up' until it will work effectively toward certain social ends" (p. 2). Bates (1976b) defined sociolinguistics as "the study of differences between social groups in the use of a given language or set of languages" (p. 452). Bates's definition of sociolinguistics is particularly appropriate for early studies which dealt with social class, race, and other differences between groups in the use of language. However, recent studies dealing with language use between twins and in mother-child interactions (Snow 1972; Clark-Stewart 1973; Nelson 1973) have also been classified as sociolinguistic. Other applications are also reported in the literature. The reader is referred to researchers such as Dittmar (1976) and Gumperz and Hymes (1972) for comprehensive discussions pertaining to sociolinguistics. This review continues with a description of major developments in pragmatics.

Major contributors to understanding children's development and use of language include Dore (1975), Halliday (1973, 1975) and Bates (1976). Dore focused on children's use of one-word utterances and defined them in terms of "speech acts" or functions, which include labeling, repeating, answering, requestioning (action), requesting (answer), calling, greeting, protesting, and practicing. Utilizing Piagetian concepts of cognitive development, Bates formulated a theory on the acquisition of pragmatic structures. The theory is comprehensive, explicating interactions among pragmatic, semantic, and syntactic systems.

Halliday described not only the functions of language during early childhood but also suggested global uses of language as the child enters adulthood. The acquisition and development of pragmatic aspects of language spans three phases according to Halliday. Phase I relates to initial uses of language, found in Halliday's single subject, Nigel, during approximately the first one and one-half years. The functions and example translations are presented in Table 3-II.

Table 3-II

Halliday's Phase I Functions of Language

Function	Example
Instrumental	I want
Regulatory	Do as I tell you
Interactional	Me and you
Personal	Here I come
Heuristic	Tell me why
Imaginative	Let's pretend
Informative	I've got something to tell you

According to Halliday, each utterance during Phase I serves only one function. However, Nigel, Halliday reported, demonstrated the informative function significantly later than the remaining functions.

Phase II marks the child's transition to adult language. Single utterances serve several functions in different grammatical contexts. During Phase II, two additional functions are exhibited: pragmatic and mathetic. The pragmatic function is derived from the instrumental and regulatory functions of Phase I and is defined as "language as doing." The mathetic function is derived from the personal and heuristic functions of Phase I and is defined as "language as learning." Ability to engage in dialogues is also developed in Phase II. The child is able to take on different roles in communicating situations, such as respondent and questioner.

Phase III is represented in adult language by two additional major functions: ideational and interpersonal. The former is defined by Halliday as the "speaker's experience and interpretation of the world that is around and inside him" (1975, p. 261). The latter function relates to the speaker's "involvement in the speech situation — his roles, attitudes, wishes, judgments, and the like" (p. 262). Also during Phase III, the textual function makes language relevant to what is said before, during, and after social interaction. The functions that language serve during Phase III are broader than the context of *use* during the early stages of language development. However, Phase III functions are derived primarily from the ideational and interpersonal functions.

The major contributors to the expanding literature on pragmatic child language are in general agreement. The consensus is that language serves ultimately to effect achievement of social interaction between the child and significant others in the environment. Each contributor in this review approaches pragmatics from a slightly different frame. But, among them, the goal of defining the functions that language serves in social interaction is achieved.

In summary, this review revealed several shifts in researchers' perspectives on children's acquisition and development of language. From stimulus-response connections and development of patterns of language behavior, the emphasis shifted to the primacy of syntax. Later it was recognized that descriptions of children's syntactical development did not account for meaning in child language. Nor did descriptions of children's syntax reveal continuity with their cognitive growth. These phenomena led to formulations of semantic grammar and descriptions of semantic relations in children's utterances. Soon it was recognized that children talk for a reason, and that the semantic relations in their utterances were context bound and served certain purposes. The cumulative result of the progressive perspectives is the recognition that components of communicative behavior — phonology, semantics, syntax, and pragmatics are interdependent. Meaningful and appropriate interactions among them account for an efficient communication system.

We turn now to issues regarding traditional evaluation and treatment of children's problems in communicative behavior. The purpose of the section is to highlight major concerns and to provide a background against which innovative approaches to language assessment-intervention may be viewed and compared.

LANGUAGE DIAGNOSIS/REMEDIATION: TRADITIONAL APPROACHES

In schools, hospitals, universities, habilitative/rehabilitative clinics, and other service delivery settings, a standard procedure for determining communication proficiency is the administration of norm referenced or standardized tests of language. Such tests have flourished during recent years; see, for example, listings by Cicciarelli, Broen and Siegel (1976), Darley and Spriestersbach (1978), and Bryne and Shervanian (1977). The tests are designed purportedly to assess various dimensions of linguistic behavior, including understanding of single words, phrases, and sentences; ability to express ideas; and aspects relative to general cognitive functioning. In most instances, the tests employ stimuli such as pictures and environmental objects to elicit responses. Scoring of the responses results in a quantification and/or classification of performance on the test. In essence, the test results enable the examiner to compare the examinee's performance with the normative sample. There are many problems inherent in this procedure as will be discussed later. At this point the discussion turns to more specific procedures in traditional diagnosis of language difficulties in autisticlike, cerebral palsied and deaf-blind children.

Diagnosis with Special Children

Traditional diagnosis of communication proficiency of children with autistic behaviors is complex. Underlying problems in development of intellectual capacity, ability to interact socially, and ability to demonstrate meaning through nonverbal and verbal codes may militate against the diagnostic procedure. In fact, the issue of whether such children are mentally retarded, mentally retarded-autistic, autistic, psychotic, or whether the primary problem is one of a generalized language deficit has not been fully resolved (Ormitz and Ritvo 1968; Wing 1966; Ricks and Wing 1975; Ritvo 1976; Rutter and Schopler 1978; deVilliers and deVilliers 1978; Bloom and Lahey 1978; Bartak and Rutter 1976). However, in psychoeducational evaluations of children with autistic behaviors, general cognitive functioning and language abilities are assessed with norm-referenced tests. Selections in the following reports are representative of the variety of tests currently utilized in many service delivery settings.

Mittler (1966) discussed psychological assessment of autistic children and recommended use of several nonverbal and verbal tests. Among nonverbal instruments, the "Three Hole Form Board" (Terman and Merrill 1960) and the "Wallin Peg Boards and Picture Puzzles from the Merrill-Palmer Scale" (Stutsman 1931) were recommended. Tests of verbal behavior included the Peabody Picture Vocabulary Test (PPVT) Dunn 1959) and several select subtests from the Illinois Test of Psycholinguistic Abilities (ITPA) (McCarthy and Kirk 1961).

Doherty and Swisher (1978) added other standardized tests for diagnostic evaluation of autistic children. They included the "Bayley Infant Intelligence Scale, WISC, Stanford-Binet, Alpern-Boll Communication Scale, Cattell-Binet, and two checklists usually filled out while interviewing the mother: Vineland Social Maturity Scale and the Alpern-Boll Self-Help Scale" (p. 554).

While the investigations of several researchers indicated use of specific standardized instruments in assessing cognitive functioning and language of children with autistic behaviors, others have developed operant-based evaluation procedures (Lovaas et al. 1965, 1972, 1974; Flaharty 1976; Frankel and Graham 1976). Further, several researchers have outlined psychoanalytic procedures for evaluating language behavior of autistic children (Bettelheim 1967; Ruttenberg 1971; Ruttenberg and Wolf 1967; Ruttenberg et al. 1966). The scope of this section will not permit full discussion of these approaches; therefore, the reader is referred to the primary sources for thorough treatment.

In summary, the literature revealed several theoretical orientations and approaches to diagnosis of language problems of children with autistic behaviors. Of the approaches noted above — psychoeducational, operant-based and psychoanalytic — the psychoeducational approach appeared to be more prevalent in a variety of service delivery settings for children with autistic behaviors. Our discussion continues with traditional language evaluation procedures with cerebral palsied children.

Many investigators have defined formidable barriers in cerebral palsied children's acquisition and development of linguistic behavior. (Mysak 1968, 1971; Phelps 1950; Marks 1974;

Safford and Arbitman 1975; Knott 1979). Among the various handicapping conditions that may affect communicative behavior in these children are mental retardation, defects in hearing, vision, perception, motor functioning, and epilepsy (Woods 1969). In reference to verbal behavior, Lencione (1968) stated that cerebral palsied children's "speech and language problems may range from very mild disorders to severe impairment dependent on the extent and range of the neuromuscular, neurosensory, and psychosensory damage" (p. 161).

Traditionally, several standardized language instruments have been administered to diagnose cerebral palsied children's language problems. As reported below, several of the tests have been delineated in descriptive studies of cerebral palsied children.

Lencione (1968) argued that "the cerebral palsied child follows the same course of linguistic development as that of the nonhandicapped child" (p. 167) and recommended several standardized language tests. For diagnostic purposes, the selection included the Verbal Language Development Scale (Mecham 1958), a "Rating Scale for Evaluation of Receptive, Expressive, and Phonetic Language Development in the Young Child" (D'Asaro and John 1961) and the ITPA. Lencione also cited "An Abstraction Test for Use with Cerebral Palsied Children" (Irwin and Hammill 1964).

DiCarlo (1974) advised that cerebral palsied children's ability to comprehend can be tested by using select items from global measures of intelligence such as the WISC and the WPPSI (Wechsler 1949, 1967). DiCarlo cautioned that items requiring verbal output to indicate comprehension should be modified so that the child is not penalized by the handicapping condition. The Vineland Social Maturity Scale (Doll 1936) was also recommended as a tool to supplement parent information about the child's communicative behavior. Numerous developmental scales described by McConnell, Love, and Clark (1974) were also recommended by DiCarlo.

Francis-Williams (1969) suggested several additional norm-referenced tests to be used in language assessment of cerebral palsied children. Familiar tests included the PPVT and the Columbia Mental Maturity Test, recently revised as a standard-

90 *Developing Assessment Programs*

ized Scale (CMMS) Burgemeister, Blum, and Lorge (1972). So far in this section the use of certain standardized language tests with children with autistic characteristics and cerebral palsied children has been addressed. The discussion continues with an examination of traditional language assessment procedures with deaf-blind children.

Jamieson (1976) and Whiting (1976) discussed general assessment of deaf-blind children, which included self-help skills, motor development, sensory, affective, and cognitive functioning. In their recommendations for selection of appropriate standardized tests to evaluate deaf-blind children's language behavior, the researchers suggested the Slingerland Specific Language Disability Test, and the Bzoch-Legue Receptive Expressive Emergent Language Scale, respectively.

Robbins (1977), describing the intent and purpose of the educational program and variables in educational assessment, listed several standardized tests used in assessing deaf-blind children. Among language measures, the author listed the Mecham Language Scales, Peabody Picture Vocabulary Test, Charles Merrill Preschool Language Scale and the Receptive-Expressive-Emergent Language Scales. Robbins also listed verbal items from the WISC and the Stanford-Binet as test tools for deaf-blind children.

As revealed in the discussion, many standardized measures of linguistic ability are currently in use with cerebral palsied, deaf-blind, and children with autisticlike behaviors. However, persistent problems and limitations are inherent in their use, particularly in describing the children's communicative behavior. The major criticism against the use of currently popular standardized language tests with exceptional children is that the tests compare exceptional children with the population of "normal" children. In this regard, sensory, developmental, and other problems manifested by exceptional children often thwart their performance, resulting in distorted scores. To date, standardized language tests are designed foremost to evaluate a child's knowledge and use of single words, phrases, and certain grammatical structures. The quantity of the items is often limited and do not relate to the child's experiences. More specifically, available language tests splinter components of communicative behavior, obviating measurement of interaction among the components and the child's use of them in situational contexts.

In addition, standardized language tests measure the child's linguistic behavior in structured or formal situations, yielding a quantification of what the child does in a given period rather than what occurs in routine situations. Following standard administration procedures, for example, adherence to time limits and one-time expression of items to the child also affects results. Similarly, when standard procedures are not followed the results from the test are not reliable (with reference to "norms.") Finally, results from standardized language tests do not assist in developing effective educational procedures. Primarily, they serve the purpose of comparing one child's performance on a test with other children.

Traditionally, following the administration of a language test or battery, the next procedure is to formulate recommendations and/or remediation strategies. Currently in special education and speech, language and hearing, and other disciplines involved with exceptional children, there is no consensus as to which language methodology is most appropriate to meet identified needs of affected children. Educational strategies vary according to experiential background, professional training, and attitudes of individuals responsible for remediation. The overall goals and objectives of administrators and other professionals may also affect selection of educational strategies. Finally, there is no shortage of language materials. In recent years, "canned" or ready-made language programs and supplementary materials have flourished. Often, criteria for development of materials to meet special needs of exceptional children are missing. No attempt is made to review the plethora of language remediation strategies and programs. The reader is referred to Dickson (1974), Lloyd (1976), and Schiefelbusch and Lloyd (1974). These researchers critique various methods and materials for language remediation.

So far in the discussion, the current state of the art in discovering language acquisition and development has been reviewed. Traditional approaches to diagnosis and remediation of children's problems in linguistic behavior have been summarized. We turn now to examine a rationale and model, representing elements of communicative behavior, on which language assessment-intervention procedures can be developed.

COMMUNICATIVE BEHAVIOR IN CHILDREN

Conceptually, the term "communication" is subject to a variety of definitions. Traditionally, however, it has been described to include two major channels for sending and receiving information: verbal and nonverbal symbolic behavior (Nolan 1975; Harper, Wiens, and Matarazzo 1978). Recently, a third dimension-context has begun to gain currency as a variant which affects expression and interpretation of verbal and nonverbal symbolic behavior (Gumperz and Hymes 1972; Bates 1976a; Moerk 1977). As such, context is regarded as a component of communicative efficiency and impairment; we continue with more specific explanations.

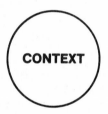

Many researchers have expressed a claim that environmental settings or contexts of verbal behavior influence meaning of children's utterances (Friedlander 1970; Greenfield and Smith 1976). The example recorded by Bloom (1970) was cited earlier in the chapter. Collectively, the researchers suggested that communication between individuals does not occur in a vacuum; it is context specific. Meanings are expressed and comprehended based on the context of the situation.

Recently, Moerk (1977) delineated communicative and formative functions of settings or contexts on verbal behavior during the early stages of language acquisition. Contexts have communicative functions in that they permit the sender of messages to encode or specify less in verbal messages. In this respect, perceptions of the context are shared between sender and receiver of messages; thus, the context serves to coordinate communication. Eliciting and structuring functions comprise formative functions of communication contexts. As Moerk explained, eliciting functions "lead to the production of previously learned verbal elements or structures but do not result in new structures" (p. 173). For example, the context may serve to enable a child to "name" objects previously experienced in the environment. Structuring functions of the communication context enable the child to go beyond direct one-to-one relations in the environment and express more complex conceptualizations based on previously acquired knowledge. The child has advanced to relate one aspect of the environment to another through various activities using verbal structures in combination with nonverbal elements or verbal structures exclusively.

Moerk related the functions of communication contexts to verbal behavior specifically and noted that similar claims for functions of communication contexts for nonverbal communication are sparsely data-based. Although empirical data are limited, a strong case for application of the principles to nonverbal symbolic behavior can be made since it is argued by many researchers that verbal and nonverbal communication are interdependent (Birdwhistell 1970; Knapp 1978). Summarizing, many aspects of the environment are shared between child and caretaker and contribute to the child's constructing an internalized view of the world. As discussed below, verbal and nonverbal symbolic behavior are instruments which are shared by caretakers and learned by the child to facilitate development, internalization of the world, and efficient communication.

Early and more contemporary researchers have asserted that ontogenetically, acquisition and development of nonverbal communication precedes comprehension and use of linguistic behavior (Piaget 1926; McCarthy 1954; Myklebust 1954; Bates 1976a; Moerk 1977). This clinical and data-based observation suggests that prior to actual sharing of communication contexts, the child establishes that acts of caretakers carry or denote meaning. Here, behavioral acts have reference to expressions of meaning through various channels of nonverbal communication. The most prominent are *proxemics* (man's perception and use of space), *paralanguage* (voice qualities accompanying spoken language), and *kinesics* (facial expressions, body movement, and gestures) (Duncan 1969).

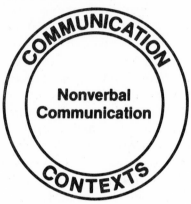

While observing behavioral acts of caretakers, the child determines that certain behavior means certain things, for example, fetching a coat signifies departure, certain movements in a kitchen indicate preparation of food. Referential meaning of these and other behavioral acts in context-specific situations are established by the child (Moerk 1977). This learning process enables the child to comprehend and use nonverbal symbolic behavior to serve directive and referential functions. According to Moerk, the behaviors are developmental in sequence. Directive behavior includes expressive gestures which result in having a desire fulfilled by a caretaker. ". . . directive messages contain in their intention structure all three basic elements of the sentence: an agent, an action, and an object" (p. 185). Referential messages are intentionally employed nonverbal symbolic behaviors, characterized by Moerk as shifting from a directive message such as "bring" to a referential message such as "look." The nonverbal messages — directive and referential — form the structural mold for later appearing verbal behavior. In this instance, the messages are performed orally instead of manually.

Besides forming the basis for future linguistic behavior, nonverbal symbolic behavior serves three communicative functions according to Moerk. Existing primarily in the form of gestural behavior, during the early years nonverbal communication functions to substitute for verbal behavior providing the child has the capacity to acquire verbal behavior. Gestures serve to complete the meaning of verbal behavior or to make verbal behavior less ambiguous. Finally, gestures serve a supportive function; they amplify certain parts of verbal behavior. Summarizing, Moerk argued that nonverbal symbolic behavior of caretakers and children and the communication context of events greatly influence the structure and content of children's early verbal behavior.

During the early stages of language acquisition, verbal and nonverbal symbolic behavior are expressed in parallel fashion.

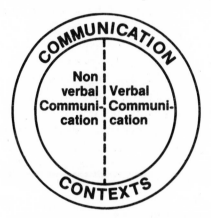

Elements of verbal language development have been described previously to include: phonological, semantic-syntax, and pragmatic aspects. As the child progresses in development of the elements, use of nonverbal symbolic decreases. However, a proportion of the message is communicated through nonverbal channels throughout adulthood. What the proportion equals in young children's communicative behavior is not known, but the significance of nonverbal communication is well recognized when we consider Birdwhistell's (1970) estimate that in any two-party adult interaction, 65 percent of the message is nonverbal.

Concluding, the interdependence of communication contexts and systems in the child's development of communicative behavior was explained. It was revealed that the child progresses developmentally from sharing the communication context with caretakers to comprehending and using nonverbal symbolic behavior. From this stage of communication development, the child advances to comprehend and use verbal behavior, however, it was also suggested that nonverbal communication comprises a portion of the message in all human interaction. At this point, the discussion turns to examine language assessment-intervention from the perspective of communicative development in young children.

LANGUAGE ASSESSMENT-INTERVENTION

Just as contextual learning is basic to language acquisition (Bloom 1970, 1973; Brown 1973; Dore 1975; Halliday 1975), it is necessary to place language assessment-intervention within a framework of context. For the purpose of determining a child's communication efficiency and needs, natural situations involving peers, parents, siblings, and others are ideal, however, near natural situations may be staged or simulated for this purpose. The objective is to obtain a description of the child's communicative behavior within and across contextual situations. The description details the child's development and use of communicative behavior, thus suggesting alternatives for improving the child's behavior through similar situations either natural or simulated.

The question arises as to how the exceptional child's communicative behavior is described. Presently, the state of knowledge about language acquisition and development is tentative; all the questions have not been answered. More important, improving exceptional children's communicative behavior cannot wait for absolutes regarding language acquisition. We must take the best available knowledge and attempt to improve children's communication ability. Further, from litigation involving exceptional children across the United States, it can be inferred that many of these children manifest language difficulties which affect academic and psychosocial performance. Much of this litigation has involved exceptional children who were previously excluded or provided only minimal service by the public schools, including cerebral palsied, deaf-blind, and children with autistic behaviors. The cases have resulted in a necessity to apply new knowledge and develop innovative approaches to communicative development and assessment intervention. To date, the improved knowledge comes from research which focuses on normal children's development of cognitive behavior, nonverbal symbolic behavior, linguistic systems, and functions of communicative behavior in social contexts. Taking as a guide the sequence of development of these components in normal developing children, a form is constructed to enable a clinician, psychologist, or educator to make observations and record systematically the behavior of children in different communication contexts. The objective is to extract patterns of interaction among the various communicative behaviors.

For the purpose of constructing a form that reflects data-based information pertinent to the sequence of development in normal children, researchers such as Bloom and Lahey (1978), McLean and Snyder-McLean (1978), Knott (1974, 1979b) and McDonald (1978) are recommended sources. Particularly, these researchers approached description of normal children's linguistic and nonlinguistic behavior from an environmental or communication-context perspective.

Having determined patterns of interaction among the components of communicative behavior in different social contexts, a child's efficiency with communicative systems is described. Procedurally, the next step is to structure activities that are conducive to fostering communicative development in context specific situations. The activities reflect the child's developmental milestones in the communicative systems, environmental stimuli familiar to the child, and how the child processes information. Muma (1978) outlined several principles from McCaffrey (1977) that should be considered conceptually in designing a "communication-based program." The principles are paraphrased from Muma (pp. 299-300).

1. ORGANIC. With respect to the components of communicative behavior, the components are not isolated as separate entities during intervention. Rather, they maintain "organic integrity" as in natural communicative behavior.
2. HUMAN. Language intervention is conducted with other individuals in various forms of social interaction.
3. MODELING. Appropriate language models are provided to

enable the child to learn language use in the manner he/she wishes to communicate.

4. PRACTICE. The child is provided various opportunities to practice language use for different communication purposes.

5. INTEGRATION. "TALKING" AND "LISTENING". Intervention strategies provide the child opportunity to function as an encoder and a decoder in social exchanges.

6. MATCH-UP. The needs of the child determine materials and activity selection.

7. FEEDBACK. As in natural communication, intervention allows the child to become aware of his message communication on others; it invites alteration of message to achieve desired effects.

8. ACCEPTANCE. Messages in natural communicative contexts are purposeful. The child's utterances should be accepted in that the aforementioned principles serve to modify utterances.

9. PRINCIPLES, PROCESSES, IDEAS. "An intervention program should be oriented on principles, processes, and ideas rather than on products . . . intervention should be about functions of language in a variety of natural contexts."

10. CHILD-TASK ORIENTATION. Flexible learning situations are created to enable the child to become an independent learner. Children cooperate in problem-solving tasks to generate solutions.

Implementation of the above principles with cerebral palsied, deaf-blind, and children with autistic behaviors as well as other language-impaired children does require consideration of developmental potential and intactness of sensory channels to receive information from the environment. Some specific considerations are discussed for cerebral palsied and deaf-blind children. A general view regarding the course of language development in children with autistic behaviors is stated.

Cerebral Palsied Children

Disturbances of auditory processes and neuromuscular development that interfere with language reception and expression are common among cerebral palsied children. Although hearing thresholds may be appropriate for normal speech and language reception, some cerebral palsied children "develop selective habits to exclude some background noise" (DiCarlo 1974). Audiological evaluations are indicated to access perception of acoustic signals and to provide instrumental assistance when appropriate. Respiratory difficulties are also characteristic of cerebral palsied children and usually affect speech intelligibility. Improvement of breathing as well as muscle coordination requires the service of a physical and/or occupational therapist. Otherwise, language assessment-intervention with cerebral palsied follows the above principles.

Deaf-Blind Children

Multiple disabilities are characteristic of deaf-blind children and require special consideration in language assessment-intervention programs. Among disabilities affecting development of communicative behavior in deaf-blind children are degree of sight and hearing, onset and progress of visual and auditory disability, movement disorders, sensitivity and arousal levels, and age of initiation of sensory aids (Robbins 1977). Not all deaf-blind children are totally impaired sensorially; peripheral vision and audition permit some children to experience normal communicative development with mild to moderate difficulty. However, other deaf-blind children are dependent on special transmission of language. Baaske (1977) listed five possible ways; (1) by feeling phonetic language from lips and larynx, (2) by means of a finger-hand alphabet, (3) by means of characters, e.g. Braille, (4) by means of natural and artificial gestures, and (5) by means of mimic and gestures. Obviously, these systems of language transmission require specialized personnel in language assessment-intervention.

Children with Autistic Behaviors

There is considerable controversy about language variation in children diagnosed as autistic or children described as manifesting autisticlike behaviors. Some researchers contend that the course of normal language development differs, however, it has not been established how and why the course of development is different. Even with the unsettled questions, several researchers' contributions to the plethora of literature on child autism support implementation of the above suggested principles for language assessment-intervention (Menyuk 1978; Lansing and Schopler 1978; Rutter 1978).

While many programs have been developed to improve communicative behavior of cerebral palsied, deaf-blind, children with autistic behaviors, and other multiply involved children, this effort represents an attempt to advance the state of the art. It has been presented with an awareness that modifications may be appropriate.

PARENT AND PROFESSIONAL ROLES

Parents

In recent years, the role of parents in the education of their exceptional children has been felt in local schools, state offices of education, and at the federal government level of the United States. Many parents of exceptional children have rejected the age-old adage that "the teacher knows best" and have assumed primary roles in their children's education through protests of school conditions, personnel, and general service delivery. This growing attitude of parents of exceptional children was reflected in their recent success in initiating legislature which resulted in the passage of Public Law 94-142, the Education for all Handicapped Children Act, 1975. The stability and political influence of exceptional children parent organizations, such as the Association for Children with Learning Disabilities and the Coordinating Council for Handicapped Children, attest to the concern of parents of exceptional children. In addition, litigation against school districts across the United States is the strongest indicator of parent interest in their children's education. Most of the litigation cases have resulted in favorable decisions for parents and their exceptional children.

Assured of entry into the public schools through P. L. 94-

142, many parents have expressed their felt needs in providing appropriate education, psychosocial experiences, physical and occupational therapy, and other services and care for their children. And, within the framework of a legal mandate, some felt needs are being met by public school and nonschool agencies. Parents of exceptional children, for example, are involved in planning their children's educational programs; they are involved in parent counseling groups related to special programs initiated by school personnel; they receive assistance in carrying out therapeutic programs in the home.

Although parents of exceptional children have been mandated the right to have active participation in their children's education, they have not assumed very active roles in specific educational programs. One reason for this is the recent acceptance of parents by professionals. Traditionally, professionals had minimal contact with parents, except for special occasions such as "open house," specially designated periods for parent-teacher conferences, or when a child disrupted the educational process. More recently, parents have been invited to assist in home-school education of their children. Many have responded to requests for information regarding their children's use of language in the home; they assist in keeping records of their children's linguistic behavior and in providing practice for language improvement. How involved parents are in assessment-intervention procedures of the type presented in this chapter is not known, however, it is suggested that parents be given every opportunity to become actively involved.

Professionals

Many professionals are involved in the education of cerebral palsied, deaf-blind, and children with autistic behaviors. They include school psychologists, speech and language clinicians, audiologists, classroom teachers, physical and occupational therapists, administrators, and others who can assist in meeting the needs of the child and the family. This interdisciplinary involvement was mandated by P. L. 94-142. With reference to language assessment-intervention, usually the school psychologist, speech and language clinician, classroom teacher, and a physical or occupational therapist, with motorically affected children are involved. Each has been designated a role in the education of all exceptional children; however, who should provide language assessment-intervention with cerebral palsied, deaf-blind children with autistic behaviors, and other multi-handicapped children in the public schools is controversial. The argument centers on the learning disabilities specialist, reading teacher, and the speech and language pathologist or language clinician. Each field has had a spokesman claim that his respective discipline deserves the responsibility. The issue is basically territoriality and economic security. The interested reader may refer to Larsen (1976), Stick (1976) for principle arguments and their suggested solutions to the problem.

The school psychologist has not been excluded from criticism in his/her role with children experiencing language impairment. The majority criticism from classroom teachers is that school psychologists have traditionally told them little they didn't already know about language problems in children. Specifically, classroom teachers have asserted that psychological reports are generally accepted to be vague in describing children's linguistic behavior. Recommendations for remediation are too telegraphic according to classroom teachers. Parents have also revealed dissatisfaction with psychologists. Many claim that the language used to describe their child's problem is not understood or they pretend understanding and then go from one source to another seeking interpretation of the psychologist's explanation. These statements reveal real concern for the integrity which currently exists between school psychologist, classroom teachers, and parents of exceptional children. With recent improvement in college and university training programs, federal funding to provide in-service training for psychologists and classroom teachers, and the recognition by school personnel that they are obligated by law to improve service delivery to exceptional children, many changes will be effected.

The proposed model for language assessment-intervention assumes participation by parents, school psychologists, classroom teachers, speech and language clinicians, and others who provide specialized sources. An interdisciplinary approach brings together possible recent trends and potential cooperation and contributions that may not be available through a single disciplinary effort.

With regard to attempts by educators to provide the best service to parents and their exceptional children, the attitudes and needs of parents of cerebral palsied (Knott 1979a), deaf-blind (Horsley 1977), and children with autistic behaviors (Wing 1966), must be taken into consideration. Often the concern for family solidarity by psychologists and classroom teachers creates less tension in the family, serves as an incentive for cooperative home-school efforts and facilitates expression of stress, fear, and anxiety, which can infringe on family dynamics.

REFERENCES

Baaske, K. H. Communication through manuals, codes, retained speech, and technical devices. *In Proceedings of the First Historic Helen Keller World Conference on Services to Deaf-Blind Youths and Adults.* Paris, World Council for the Welfare of the Blind, 1977.

Barker, L., and Kibler, R. (Eds.) *Speech Communication Behavior.* Englewood Cliffs, New Jersey, P-H, 1971.

Bartak, L., and Rutler, M. Differences between mentally retarded and normally intelligent autistic children. *J Autism Child Schizophr, 6*(2): 109-120, 1976.

Bates, E. *Language and Context: The Acquisition of Pragmatics.* New York., Acad Pr, 1976(a).

Bates, E. Pragmatics and sociolinguistics in child language. In Moorehead, D., and Moorehead, A. (Eds.): *Normal and Deficient Child Language.* Baltimore, Univ Park, 1976(b).

Bettelheim, B. *The Empty Fortress: Infantile Autism and the Birth of the Self.* New York, Free Pr, 1967.

Birdwhistell, R. *Kinesics and Context.* Philadelphia, U of Pa Pr, 1970.

Bloom, L. *Language Development: Form and Function in Emerging Grammars.* Cambridge, Massachusetts, MIT Pr, 1970.

Bloom, L. Why not pivot grammar? *J. Speech Hear Disord, 36:* 40-50, 1971.

Bloom, L. *One Word at a Time: The Use of Single-Word Utterances Before Syntax.* The Hague, Mouton, 1973.

Bloom, L., and Lahey, M. *Language Development and Language Disorders.* New York, Wiley, 1978.

Bowerman, M. Structural relationships in children's utterances: Syntactic or semantic? In Moore, T. E. (Ed.) *Cognitive Development and the Acquisition of Language.* New York, Acad Pr, 1973.

Brown, R. *A First Language: The Early Stages.* Cambridge, Massachusetts, Harvard U Pr. 1973.

Brown, R.; Cazden, C.; and Bellugi, U. The child's grammar from one to three. In Hill, J. P. (Ed.) *Minnesota Symposium on Child Psychology.* Minneapolis, U of Minn Pr, 1969, vol. II.

Bruner, J. From communication to language — a psychological perspective. *Cognition, 3:* 255-288, 1975.

Burgemeister, B.; Blum, L.; and Lorge, I. Columbia Mental Maturity Scale, 3rd ed. New York, Har Brace J, 1972.

Bryne, M., and Shervanian, C. *Introduction to Communicative Disorders.* New York, Har-Row, 1977.

Carrow, M. The development of auditory comprehension of language structure in children. *J Speech Hear Disord, 33:* 99-111, 1968.

Chomsky, N. *Syntactic Structures.* The Hague, Mouton, 1957.

Chomsky, N. *Aspects of a Theory of Syntax.* Cambridge, Massachusetts, MIT Pr, 1965.

Chomsky, N., and Halle, M. *The Sound Pattern of English.* New York, Har-Row, 1968.

Cicciarelli, A.; Broen, P.; and Siegel, G. Language assessment procedures, Appendix A. In Lloyd, L. L. (Ed.); *Communication Assessment and Intervention Strategies.* Baltimore, Univ Park, 1976.

Clark-Stewart, K. Interactions between mothers and their young children: Characteristics and consequences. Society for Research in Child Development. Monograph No. 153, 1973.

Darley, F., and Spriestersbach, D. *Diagnostic Methods in Speech Pathology,* 2nd ed. New York, Har-Row, 1978.

D'Asaro, M., and John, V. Rating scale for evaluation of receptive, expressive and phonetic language development in the young child. *Cerebral Palsy Review, 22:* 3-4, 1961.

deVilliers, J., and deVilliers, P. *Language Acquisition.* Cambridge, Massachusetts, Harvard U Pr, 1978.

DiCarlo, L. Communication therapy for problems associated with cerebral palsy. In Dickson, S. (Ed.): *Communication Disorders: Remedial Principles and Practices.* Glenview, Illinois, Scott F, 1974.

Dickson, S. *Communication disorders: Remedial Principles and Practices.* Glenview, Illinois, Scott F, 1974.

Dittmar, N. *Sociolinguistics: A Critical Survey of Theory and Application.* London, Arnold, 1976.

Doherty, L., and Sivisher, L. Children with autistic behaviors. In Minifie, F. and Lloyd, L. (Eds.): *Communicative and Cognitive Abilities — Early Behavioral Assessment.* Baltimore, Univ Park, 1978.

Doll, E. *Vineland Social Maturity Scale.* Minneapolis, Am Guidance, 1936.

Dore, J. Holophrases, speech arts and language universals. *Journal of Child Language, 2:* 21-40, 1975.

Duncan, S. Nonverbal communication. *Psychol Bull, 72:* 118-137, 1969.

Dunn, L. *The Peabody Picture Vocabulary Test.* Minneapolis, Am Guidance,

1959.

Ferguson, C., and Garnica, O. Theories of phonological development. In Lenneberg, E., and Lenneberg, E. (Eds.): *Foundations of Language Development.* New York, Acad Pr, 1975, vol. I.

Fillmore, C. The case for case. In Bach, E., and Harms, R. (Eds.): *Universal in Linguistic Theory.* New York, HR&W, 1968.

Flaharty, R. Preschool assessment. In Retvo, E. (Ed.) *Autism: Diagnosis, Current Research and Management.* New York, Spectrum, 1976.

Foss, D., and Hakes, D. Psycholinguistics: An Introduction to the Psychology of Language. Englewood Cliffs, New Jersey, P-H, 1978.

Francis-Williams, J. Assessment of cerebral palsied children: A survey of advances since 1958. In Wolf, J., and Anderson, R. (Eds.): *The Multiply Handicapped Child.* Springfield, Thomas, 1969.

Frankel, F., and Graham, V. Systematic observation of classroom behavior of retarded and autistic preschool children. Am *J of Ment Defic, 81*(1): 73-84, 1976.

Friedlander, B. Receptive language development in infancy: Issues and problems. *Merrill Palmer Quarterly, 16:* 7-51, 1970.

Greenfield, P., and Smith, J. *The Structure of Communication in Early Language Development.* New York, Acad Pr, 1976.

Greene, J. *Psycholinguistics: Chomsky and Psychology.* Baltimore, Penguin, 1972.

Gumperz, J., and Hymes, D. (Eds.). *Directions in Sociolinguistics.* New York, HR&W, 1972.

Halliday, M. A. K. *Explorations in the Functions of Language.* London, Arnold, 1973.

Halliday, M. A. K. Learning how to mean. In Lenneberg, E., and Lenneberg, E. (Eds.): Foundations of Language Development: A Multidisciplinary Approach. New York, Acad Pr, 1975, vol. I.

Harper, R.; Wiens, A.; and Matarazzo, J. *Nonverbal Communication: The State of the Art.* New York, Wiley, 1978.

Horsley, J. Home visitation and counseling. In Lowell, E., and Rouin, C. (Eds.). *State of the Art: Perspectives on Serving Deaf-Blind Children.* Sacramento, California State Department of Education, 1977.

Ingram, D. *Phonological Disability in Children.* New York, Elsevier, 1976.

Irwin, J., and Marge, M. (Eds.). *Principles of Childhood Language Disabilities.* New York, ACC, 1972.

Irwin, O., and Hammill, D. An abstraction test for use with cerebral palsied children. *Cerebral Palsy Review, 25:* 3-9, 1964.

Jamieson, F. Psychological implications for assessing the deaf-blind. In Rouin, C.: *Proceedings: Rubella Deaf-Blind Child: Implications of Psychological Assessment.* Sacramento, California State Department of Education, 1976.

Knapp, M. *Nonverbal Communication in Human Interaction,* 2nd ed. New York, HR&W, 1978.

Knott, G. A Study of Gesture as Nonverbal Communication in Preschool

Language Disabled and Preschool Normal Children. Unpublished Doctoral Dissertation, 1974, Northwestern University, Evanston, Illinois.

Knott, G. Attitudes and needs of parents of cerebral palsied children. *Rehab Lit, 40*(7): 190-195, 206, 1979a.

Knott, G. Nonverbal communication during early childhood. *Theory into Practice, 16*(4): 226-233, 1979b.

Lahey, M. (Ed.). *Readings in Childhood Language Disorders.* New York, Wiley, 1978.

Lakoff, R. Language in context. *Language, 48*: 907-927, 1972.

Lansing, M., and Schopler, E. Individualized education: A Public school model. In Rutter, M., and Schopler, E. (Eds.): *Autism: A Reappraisal of Concepts and Treatment.* New York, Plenum Pub, 1978.

Larsen, S. The learning disabilities specialist: Roles and responsibilities. *Journal of Learning Disabilities, 9*(8), 1976.

Lee, L. Developmental sentence scoring: A clinical procedure for estimating syntactic development in children's spontaneous speech. *J. Speech Hear Disord, 36*: 315-338, 1971.

Lencione, R. A rationale for speech and language evaluation in cerebral palsy. *Br J Disord Commun 3*(1): 161-170, 1968.

Lloyd, L. (Ed.). *Communication Assessment and Intervention Strategies.* Baltimore, Univ Park, 1976.

Lovaas, O.; Freitzg, G.; Gold, V.; and Kassorla, I. Recording apparatus and procedure for observation of behaviors of children in free play settings. *J Exp Child Psychol, 2*: 108-120, 1965.

Lovaas, O.; Koegel, R.; Simmons, J.: Long, J.; and Stevens, J. Some generalizations and 'follow-up measures on autistic children in behavior therapy. *J Appl Behav Anal, 6*: 131-166, 1972.

Lovaas, O.; Schriebman, L.; and Koegel, R. A behavior modification approach to the treatment of autistic children. *J Autism Child Schizophr, 4*: 111-129, 1974.

McCaffrey, A. Talking in class: a non-didactic approach to oral language in the elementary classroom. *Quebec Francais, 25*, 1977.

McCarthy, D. Language development in children. In Carmichael, L. (Ed.): *Manual of Child Psychology,* 2nd ed. New York, Wiley, 1954.

McCarthy, J., and Kirk, S. *The Illinois Test of Psycholinguistic Abilities.* Exp. ed. Urbana, Illinois, U of Ill Pr, 1961.

McConnell, F.; Love, R.; and Clark, B. Language remediation in children. In Dickson, S. (Ed.): *Communication Disorders: Remedial Principles and Practices.* Glenview, Illinois, Scott F, 1974.

McDonald, J. *Parent-Administered Communication Inventory.* Columbus, Ohio, Merrill, 1978.

McLean, J., and Snyder-McLean, L. *A Transactional Approach to Early Language Training.* Columbus, Ohio, Merrill, 1978.

McNeill, D. *The Acquisition of Language: The Study of Developmental Psycholinguistics.* New York, Har-Row, 1970.

Marks, N. *Cerebral Palsied and Learning Disabled Children.* Springfield, Thomas, 1974.

Mecham, M. *Verbal Language Development Scale.* Minnesota, Educational Test Bureau, 1958.

Menyuk, P. *The Acquisition and Development of Language.* Englewood Cliffs, New Jersey, P-H, 1971.

Menyuk, P. Language: What's wrong and why. In Rutter, M., and Schopler, E. (Eds.): *Autism: A Reappraisal of Concepts and Treatment.* New York, Plenum Pub, 1978.

Mittler, P. The psychological assessment of autistic children. In Wing, J. K. (Ed.). *Early Childhood Autism: Clinical, Educational and Social Aspects.* New York, Pergamon, 1966.

Moerk, E. *Pragmatics and Semantic Aspects of Early Language Development.* Baltimore, Univ Park, 1977.

Moorehead, D., and Moorehead, A. (Eds.). *Normal and Deficient Child Language.* Baltimore, Univ Park, 1976.

Muma, J. *Language Handbook: Concepts, Assessment, Intervention.* Englewood Cliffs, New Jersey, P-H, 1978.

Myklebust, H. R. *Auditory disorders in children.* New York. Grune, 1954.

Mysak, E. *Neuroevolutional approach to cerebral palsy and speech.* New York, Tchrs Coll, 1968.

Mysak, E. Cerebral palsy speech habilitation. In Travis, L. (Ed.): *Handbook of Speech Pathology and Audiology.* Englewood Cliffs, New Jersey, P-H, 1971.

Nelson, K. Structure and strategy in learning to talk. *Monogr Soc Res Child Dev, 38, (Serial No. 149)*, 1973.

Nolan, M. The relationship between verbal and nonverbal communication. In Hanneman, G. and McEwen, W. (Eds.): *Communication and Behavior.* Reading, Massachusetts, A-W, 1975.

Ornitz, E., and Ritvo, E. Perceptual inconstancy in early infantile autism: The syndrome of early infant autism and its variants including certain cases of childhood schizophrenia. *Arch Gen Psychiatry, 18*: 76-98, 1968.

Phelps, W. Etiology and diagnostic classification of cerebral palsy. In Abbott, M. (Ed.): *Proceedings of the Cerebral Palsy Institute.* New York, Association for the Aid of Crippled Children, 1950.

Piaget, J. *The Language and Thought of the Child.* London, Routledge & Kegan, 1926.

Piaget, J. *The Psychology of Intelligence.* New York, Har Brace, 1950.

Postal, P. The best theory. In Peters, S. (Ed.): *Goals in Linguistics.* Englewood Cliffs, New Jersey, P-H, 1972.

Raven, J. *Guide to Using the Coloured Progressive Matrices.* London, Lewis, 1965.

Ricks, D., and Wing, L. Language, communication, and use of symbols in normal and autistic children. *J Autism Child Schizophr, 5*(3), 191-221, 1975.

Ritvo, E. (Ed.). *Autism: Diagnosis, Current Research and Management.* New

York, Spectrum Pub, 1976.
Robbins, N. Educational assessment of deaf-blind and auditorily visually impaired children: A survey. In Lowell, E., and Rouin, C. (Eds.): *State of the Art: Perspectives on Serving Deaf-Blind Children.* Sacramento, California State Department of Education, 1977.
Ruttenberg, B. A psychoanalytic understanding of infantile autism and its treatment. In Churchill, D.; Alpern, G.; and DeMyer, M. (Eds.): *Infantile Autism.* Springfield, Thomas, 1971.
Ruttenberg, B.; Dratman, M.; Fraknoi, J.; and Wenar, C. An instrument for evaluating autistic children. *J Am Acad Child Psychiatry,* 5: 453-78, 1966.
Ruttenberg, B., and Wolf, E. Evaluating the communication of the autistic child. *J Speech Hear Disord, 32:* 314-324, 1967.
Rutter, M. Language disorder and infantile autism. In Rutter, M., and Schopler, E. (Eds.): *Autism: A Reappraisal of Concepts and Treatment.* New York, Plenum Pub, 1978.
Rutter, M., and Schopler, E. (Eds.). *Autism: A Reappraisal of Concepts and Treatment.* New York, Plenum Pub, 1978.
Safford, P., and Arbitman, D. *Developmental Intervention with Young Physically Handicapped Children.* Springfield, Thomas, 1975.
Schiefelbusch, R. (Ed.). *Bases of Language Intervention.* Baltimore, Univ Park, 1978.
Schiefelbusch, R., and Lloyd, L. (Eds.). *Language Perspective — Acquisition, Retardation, and Intervention.* Baltimore, Univ Park, 1974.
Schlesinger, I. Production of utterances and language acquisition. In Slobin, D. (Ed.): *The Ontogenesis of Grammar.* New York, Acad Pr, 1971.
Snow, C. Mother's speech to children learning language. *Child Dev, 43:* 549-566, 1972.
Stick, S. The speech pathologist and handicapped learners. *Journal of Learning Disabilities, 9*(8), 1976.
Stutsman, R. *Mental Measurement of Pre-School Children.* New York, World Books, 1931.
Terman, L., and Merrill, M. *Revised Stanford-Binet Intelligence Scale,* 3rd ed. Boston, H-M, 1960.
Wallace, G. Interdisciplinary efforts in learning disabilities: Issues and recommendations. *Journal of Learning Disabilities, 9*(8), 1976.
Wechsler, D. *Wechsler Intelligence Scale for Children.* New York, Psych Corp, 1949.
Wechsler, D. *Wechsler Preschool and Primary Scale of Intelligence.* New York, Psych Corp, 1967.
Whiting, C. Assessment of the deaf-blind child in the public school. In Rouin, C. *Proceedings: Rubella Deaf-Blind Child: Implications of Psychological Assessment.* Sacramento, California State Department of Education, 1976.
Wiig, E., and Semel, E. *Language Disabilities in Children and Adolescents.* Columbus, Ohio, Merrill, 1976.

Wing, J. (Ed.). *Early Childhood Autism: Clinical, Educational and Social Aspects.* New York, Pergamon, 1966.

Winitz, H. *Articulatory Acquisition and Behavior.* Englewood Cliffs, New Jersey, P-H, 1969.

Woods, G. The medical aspect of cerebral palsy. *Br J Disord Commun,* 4(1): 26-32, 1969.

CHAPTER FOUR

ASSESSMENT GUIDELINES FOR THE HEARING IMPAIRED

ROBERT ROBINSON, PH.D.

TESTING THE DEAF

AS is true for many other types of handicapped populations, there are simply not enough instruments devised for or standardized on the deaf to cover the many needs and situations that call for valid test information. As a result of this impoverishment, testers of the deaf often supplement their slim resources by dipping into the pool of measures that have been standardized on the hearing. However, it should be recognized that the deaf child's world is a place of widely differing sensory, perceptual, and associated life experiences from those of the hearing. Consequently, the practice of assessing deaf children by means of norms and test-items devised for the hearing results in a situation that is often unfair for both the child and examiner. The child is evaluated on a biased frame of reference, and the examiner is deprived of direct access to the evaluative system needed for objective assessment. In view of these practices, the extent to which standardized tests can be altered, as well as the implications for appropriate test selection for examiners of deaf children, need to be carefully examined.

Appropriate Test Selection

Applying good test selection procedures to deaf children calls for a rigorous study in-depth and detail of test assets and limitations. In fact, one of the cardinal rules in this regard is that an examiner does not use a test without knowing it and using it beforehand.

Besides proper standardization, there are many factors involved in choosing a particular test for a given subject. Perhaps

110

the most important single factor concerns the items of which the test is composed. For example, items in intelligence tests are selected to elicit responses that measure mental ability. Mental ability, in turn, is composed of various mental processes. What the mental processes themselves add up to is a sampling of mental behaviors that these constructors consider representative of their concept of intelligence.

Similarly, because some tests have a wide range of items and others are very narrow in scope or essentially comprised of one kind of item or task, it is very important that a matching procedure be conducted whereby there will be maximal relatedness between the individual's particular background of experiences and the items to which he will be responding. Also, there should be minimal interference with comprehension of test directions, expression of response, and general adherence to test rationale.

Another point of importance concerning test items lies in their construction. Each item of a standardized test actually is, in itself, a unit task with its own separate norm and score performance. Thus, in utilizing the results of intelligence tests in a meaningful way, a careful analysis needs to be made of the individual's level of response to each item of the test scale. Again, to accomplish this it is necessary to know what mental processes the individual items are measuring. This information can generally be found in the test constructor's standardization description. If not, the examiner must unravel it for himself. In any event, without this analysis the IQ by itself would be a fairly meaningless bit of information.

Still another point to keep in mind with regard to intellectual assessment and test selection is that different types of tests probe different aspects of intelligence. Since one of the primary aims in testing deaf children is to make as comprehensive an intellectual assessment as possible, the use of test batteries is the recommended procedure. In other words, the major purpose and immediate concern should be to determine the kinds of training and experiences that will best promote the child's functional-adaptive abilities rather than to predict whether the child will eventually be able to compete successfully with his age peers. The type of battery recommended for this purpose should consist of a performance test, a paper and pencil test, and one or more of the single-item tests such as mazes or figure drawings. Another argument for the use of the battery approach lies in the fact that doubts have increasingly been expressed concerning the value of manipulative formboard materials, traditionally used in the testing of deaf children, as indicators of intelligence. In support of this statement, Wechsler (1944) states that such materials turn out to be poor indicators of intelligence when checked against clinical experience. It should also be remembered that whenever test scales are used that consist of a verbal portion and a performance portion, such as the Wechsler scales, the use of the performance portion alone is actually the use of only half of the test and the examiner is getting only half the mental coverage. The implication here again is that it is important that such test findings be supplemented by data from other sources.

A final argument for comprehensive and diversified testing procedures is that objective testing provides but one kind of contribution, namely, information obtained under standardized conditions. This information by itself is rarely sufficient to provide the whole picture. To obtain a more complete understanding of the child as a total functioning organism requires not only the use of a battery of tests, but a number of other evaluative approaches such as: direct observation and behavior rating, life history method, interview, and introspective reporting. Further, these evaluative approaches used by themselves are nothing more than sophisticated information-gathering devices. More important is how the pooled information is used. This, of course, depends upon the skills of the examiner in collecting the data, integrating information from diverse sources, and interpreting the whole.

Test Modifications

In order to make standardized tests applicable to handicapped children, various modifications in administration and/or testing procedures have been advocated. While it is not likely that certain modifications in standard procedures will produce equivalent results, it is important to know to what extent the modified procedures yield results similar to them. For example, Strother (1945) points out that modifications in test stimuli are likely to alter the nature of the item and, consequently, the validity and reliability of the item may be affected. Braen and Masling (1959) also suggest that omitting certain subtests which require abilities not possessed by the child lead to problems associated with reliability and validity. Graham and Shapiro (1953) found that in a group of normal children between the ages of six years three months and twelve years and two months, pantomime instructions led to significantly lower WISC performance scores than did standard instructions. Sattler (1970) states that while significant group differences may not appear under modified and standard procedures, individual subjects may show large differences under the two procedures. He, therefore, suggests that new norms be developed that are based upon scores obtained under modified procedures for both normal and handicapped populations.

In general, little is known about the effects of modifications on obtained test results. Blum, Burgemeister, and Lorge (1951) point out that in using modifications there is insufficient attention paid to cross-checking the results with those of normal children. McCarthy (1958) also states the problem is in determining what normal children do with the same modified tasks.

The little research evidence that has been produced reveals conflicting findings with regard to utilizing modified testing procedures in assessing handicapped children. The majority of the findings suggest, however, that modifying test procedures does not necessarily produce significant changes in performance (Vernon and Brown 1964).

In spite of difficulties with test modification procedures, it is still important to compare the deaf child's performance with that of the normal child. This is important not only for purposes of educational and vocational planning, but because the deaf live in the same world as the hearing, and the latter sets the standards of the world at large.

Whenever a test has been standardized for pantomime directions, modification is not required when used with the deaf. The problem arises in regard to verbal instructions, which usually call for modifications, i.e. ways to make the test direc-

tions comprehensible to the subject. Levine (1971) states that
with proper care and effort, modifications can be made without
harming the original intent and objectivity of administration.
However, where modifications have been undertaken, they
should be worked out beforehand with objective directions prepared in three main forms: simplified verbal language, signs,
and pantomime. The particular form used depends upon
which is most comprehensible to the subject.

Research Needs

Despite the fact that intelligence tests are used so much in
investigations of the deaf, there is a critical shortage of tests
standardized on deaf populations. As a result, there is a crucial
need for in-depth psychological instruments standardized on a
broad chronological range of the deaf population.

In summary, the most pressing research needs in psychological assessment for the deaf, as reported by Harris (1950), are as
follows: (1) More nonverbal instruments are needed to determine how the conceptualization, abstract thinking, and
learning processes are similar to and different from the same
processes in hearing persons. Such instruments could be used
to study these processes from the very young child to the adult.
(2) Existing tests need two sets of norms: norms on the hearing
population and norms on the deaf population. Such instruments and norms could then be used more effectively for educational and vocational guidance and placement. (3) Instruments
need to be constructed and standardized that will permit the
measurement and prediction of the deaf person's capacity to
learn by the various methods of communication now used:
speech, speechreading, fingerspelling, and the language of
signs. (4) More attention should be given to ways and means of
combining the skills of many individuals in a number of disciplines in the area of psychological assessment.

Review of Test Instruments for the
Deaf and Hearing Impaired

The following section includes a review of various assessment instruments that are appropriate in testing the deaf and hearing impaired. These instruments have been categorized under five major domains for the reader's convenience and represent an up-to-date listing of instrumentation available for the deaf and hearing impaired: Intellectual Assessment, Language Skills, Motor-Perceptual Development, Self-Help, and Social-Affective.

ASSESSMENT GUIDELINES
Deaf and Hearing Impaired

I. Intellectual Assessment

A. Leiter International Performance Scale

   1. Purpose: Nonverbal test of general intelligence for deaf or speech impaired.

   2. Description: Scale consists of 54 tests ranging in difficulty from 2 to 18 years. Types of tasks range from matching colors and forms to completion of patterns, analogous designs and classification of objects.

   3. Administration: Individual — no time limit. Directions are pantomimed.

   4. Technical Data: There is a lack of reliability data and standard deviations reported for various age levels. Manual also fails to describe the standardization group. Studies have shown that the Leiter correlates in the moderate to high range with the Binet.

   5. Additional Comments: Most of the items require a good deal of perceptual organization and discrimination. Certain pictures are outdated. There is a relatively small number of test items which represent each year level. Also, item difficulty levels appears to be uneven at each year level. Norms tend to underestimate the child's intelligence. As a result, Leiter recommends that five points be added to the obtained IQ score.

   6. Publisher: Stoelling Company

1350 South Kostner Avenue
Chicago, IL 60623

B. Kahn Intelligence Test

1. Purpose: To measure intelligence of subjects who are verbally or culturally handicapped. Also has a scale for use with the deaf and blind.

2. Description: Test items for this age scale, which extend from 1 month to adulthood, are patterned after those of the Gesell Developmental Schedules and the Stanford Binet Intelligence Scale. Covers a wide range of areas.

3. Administration: Individually administered. The test requires understanding of language but few verbal responses. Can be administered by sign language to accommodate the deaf.

4. Technical Data: Kahn reports a test-retest reliability of .94 based on the MAs of 23 children ranging in age from 1 to 14 years. Validity is based on correlations of MAs on the KIT and Stanford Binet. Correlations from two different studies range from .75 to .83.

5. Additional Comments: Test instructions become complex at older ages. Although the KIT consists of interesting material and has good promise, it should be used with caution until it has been better standardized (standardized only 40 adults and 297 children).

6. Publisher: Psychological Tests Specialists
Box 1441
Missoula, MT 59801

C. Peabody Picture Vocabulary

1. Purpose: To provide a quick estimate of the individual's verbal intelligence through receptive knowledge of vocabulary.

2. Description: Consists of 150 plates with 4 pictures on each plate. Plates are arranged in difficulty from 1 year 9 months to 13 years.

3. Administration: Individually administered. Responses are nonoral. Testing ranges from 10 to 15 minutes. For deaf children, it is possible to present the Peabody by typing the words on the cards rather than presenting them orally.

4. Technical Data: Studies indicate the Peabody has adequate concurrent validity. Correlations between the Peabody and Binet range from .22 to .92 with a median correlation of .66. Alternate form reliability is reported at each age level and ranges from .67 to .84. Norms were restricted to Nashville, Tennessee population.

5. Additional Comments: Peabody score should never be considered in isolation of other measures of intelligence and should never be considered interchangeable with Binet or WISC results. Caution needs to be exercised in interpreting norms, particularly with minority or ethnic groups.

6. Publisher: American Guidance Service, Inc.
Publishers' Building
Circle Pines, MN 55014

D. Sniders-Oomen Non-Verbal Intelligence Tests for Deaf and

Hearing Subjects

1. Purpose:	To sample four aspects of intelligence: form, combination, abstraction, and memory. Appropriate for ages 3 to 16.
2. Description:	Scale includes 9 scores: mosaic, picture memory, arrangement, analogies, completion, Knox cubes, drawing, sorting, and individual IQ. Each subtest forms a separate point scale. Tables are provided to convert scores into deviation IQ.
3. Administration:	Can be administered orally or in pantomime. Individually administered.
4. Technical Data:	Reliability is reported as split-half coefficients for whole scale at ages 5 to 5 1/2 years, 10 to 11 years, and 15 years. Validity as a measure of intelligence is based on teachers' judgments. A group of 78 deaf pupils was tested in 1952 and again in 1956. Correlations of the two sets of scores with teachers' judgments made in 1956 were .42 and .49 respectively. These are .94 and .91 respectively, for hearing children and .95, .93, and .94 for deaf children. Reliability figures for the separate subtests vary from .36 to .93.
5. Additional Comments:	Appears to be a well-constructed scale. In structure it has the advantage over various Binet revisions in that its pattern is the same at all ages. Also, is a point scale rather than age scale. How-

ever, standardization sample included Dutch children only.

6. Publisher: J. B. Wolters
                             Groninger, Holland

E. Progressive Matrices (Raven)

1. Purpose: A test which attempts to estimate the general level of intellectual functioning of individuals who have communication disorders.

2. Description: The tasks consist of 60 perceptual problems which require discerning some meaningful relationships. The tasks become progressively more difficult. The scale is intended to cover the whole range of intellectual development from the time a child is able to grasp the idea of finding a missing place to the point where he can solve the whole problem.

3. Administration: Scale can be individually administered, self-administered, or given to a group. Tests are easy to administer and are brief.

4. Technical Data: Norms are available only for 1947 test. Reliability ranges from .76 to .91. Standardized on British subjects only.

5. Additional Comments: The clinical usefulness of the Matrices is limited. It is impossible to determine from the subject's attempts to deal with the tasks what he is thinking when he is wrong. Tests seem to provide a measure of perceptual adequacy rather than of intellectual capacity. According to authorities, the test does not do as good

a job as the Leiter Scale in tapping the individual's process of thinking.

6. Publisher: The Psychological Corporation
304 East 45th Street
New York, NY 10017

F. Hiskey-Nebraska Test of Learning Aptitude

1. Purpose: Assesses general intelligence or aptitude for academic achievement for deaf children 3 to 16 years of age.

2. Description: Consists of 12 subtests that tap the major psychological components necessary in school learning of deaf children. This includes: picture identification and association, visual attention span, memory for digits and colors, bead patterns, paper folding, puzzle blocks, picture analogies and completion of drawings to name a few.

3. Administration: Individually administered. Takes approximately 45 to 60 minutes.

4. Technical Data: Reliability (split-half) reported .95 for deaf population and .93 for normal hearing in age group 11 to 17. Validity is reported in terms of correlation of HNTLA IQs with Stanford Binet and WISC scores for subjects ranging in age 3 to 10 years. For Stanford Binet a correlation of .86 is reported. For WISC, correlation between IQs is .82.

5. Additional Comments: Appears to be a promising test for assessing the learning capabilities of the deaf. The behavior samplings in the areas of mem-

ory, picture identification, and picture association in particular have demonstrated relevance to the kinds of learning aptitude important in school work.

6. Publisher: Marshall S. Hiskey
                        5640 Baldwin
                        Lincoln, NE 68507

G. Merrill-Palmer Scale of Mental Tests

1. Purpose: A preschool mental test constructed to serve as a substitute for, or supplement to, revisions of the Binet Scale. Suitable for the hearing impaired.

2. Description: This scale is composed of 3 to 14 test items per six-month age period beginning at 18 months and extending to 6 years. The majority of items depend in part on fine motor skill: pegboard, block building, tower building, drawing, form board, etc. There are a few verbal items which can be omitted. This is taken into consideration in arriving at a mental age.

3. Administration: Testing begins at the age group in which the child's chronological age falls, unless he is over 47 months old, then testing should begin with the 48 to 53 month test. Each test is given completely once only. If the child passes at one level, he automatically passes at the lower levels. If a child passes more than one-half of the test at any one age group, then tests at the next age group are administered. If the

	child fails any one age group, then tests at preceding age group are administered.
4. Technical Data:	The reliability of the scale is not reported in the manual, but the author states that the test is valid on the basis that it is composed of items which differentiate between children judged bright and dull by other criteria and yields high correlations with chronological age as well as with Stanford Binet mental ages.
5. Additional Comments:	One of the major faults of the scale is that a large proportion of the tests are timed. Thus, the slow moving, but thoughtful child is penalized. Another difficulty is the scores which the scale yields. The standard deviations of the mental ages do not increase in proportion to advancing chronological ages so that IQs cannot be computed.
6. Publisher:	C. H. Stoelting Company 424 N. Homan Avenue Chicago, IL 60624

H. Arthur Point Scale of Performance Test

1. Purpose:	A non-verbal intelligence scale suitable for assessing deaf children, delayed speech, and other handicapped persons in the verbal area from ages 4 years 5 months to 15 years 5 months.
2. Description:	Instrument consists of two forms, Forms I and II. Form II is designed for retest purposes only. Test consists of five subtests, each separately standard-

ized and combined into a single point scale.

3. Administration: Is individually administered. Materials provided are convenient and easy to use, and directions are adequate.

4. Technical Data: Norms are based on 968 middle-class subjects. Adequate data on reliability and validity have not been presented by the author.

5. Additional Comments: Further validation studies are needed. Norms also need to be expanded to include minority group representation.

6. Publisher: Form I C. H. Stoelting Company
1350 S. Kostner Avenue
Chicago, IL 60623
Form II Psychological Corporation
304 E. 45th Street
New York, NY 10017

I. The Porteus Maze Test

1. Purpose: A performance test of intelligence yielding test age scores which may be converted into IQ estimates.

2. Description: The materials consist of three different maze series: The core set of 12 mazes and two extension forms, each consisting of eight mazes. Test is entirely nonverbal and provides three scores: (1) Ability Score, which indicates degree of success in solving problems; (2) Q-Score, which indicates style of response, i.e. impulsiveness, carelessness, and (3) Conformity-Variability Score.

3. Administration: Even though directions are verbal, it is possible to circumvent the use of spoken language. Test is simple and is based on individual's ability to thread his way through various mazes. Behaviors called for in this test are: recognition of the goal, identification of subgoals, short-term memory, and carry-out a plan of action.

4. Technical Data: Although maze ability scores have been found to correlate well with a variety of ability tests, the Porteus Maze Test is lacking in sufficient information on reliability, norms, and other pertinent information.

5. Additional Comments: While having good promise, the full development of the test's potential has suffered from a lack of clearly focused validation research. Test has good potential in diagnosing brain damage.

6. Publisher: George G. Harrap and Company, Ltd.
182 High Holborn
London, England

ASSESSMENT GUIDELINES
Deaf and Hearing Impaired

II. Language Skills

A. Deaf-Blind Program and Ability Screening Test

1. Purpose: Designed to determine the individual functioning and program needs of persons with multiple handicaps.

2. Description: Test assesses functioning in seven developmental areas including communication. Has been prepared for use by teachers and other professionals working with deaf-blind children. The underlying rationale for this test is based on Gessell's Developmental Theory.

3. Administration: This is an individual screening test that is mostly scored by general observation of the child. However, rattlers, blocks, and small items will be used in several test items. Test is short and requires only about 10 minutes to complete.

4. Technical Data: Adequate measures of reliability and validity have not been established as yet. Has also been standardized on small population samples.

5. Additional Comments: Interpretations from utilization of this test should be based on the consideration that formal reliability and validity measures are lacking. However, test does seem to yield practical and useful kinds of information.

6. Publisher: Mississippi Deaf-Blind-
Evaluation Center
Ellisville State School
Ellisville, Mississippi 39437

B. Diagnostic Test of Speechreading

1. Purpose: A diagnostic procedure for evaluating the deaf child's ability to comprehend the spoken word.

2. Description: This test is filmed and consists of two cartridges, each requiring three and one-half minutes of running time. The first cartridge consists of the word portions while the second cartridge contains the phrases and sentences portions. In addition to the film, the test includes 64 plates made up of 4 pictures each. The test also includes 3 plates for use in demonstrating what the child being tested is to do. Appropriate for ages 4 to 9 years.

3. Administration: The test was filmed so that each item appears twice; the item is spoken and then repeated. A time interval between each item permits the examiner to stop the projector and record the response. There is no time limit as the examiner judges when the child has had sufficient time to indicate his choice.

4. Technical Data: The test was standardized on 60 children at 3 different age levels. Subjects were of normal intelligence, but with a pure-tone hearing loss of 75dB or greater on the better ear. Reliability is established by the intercorrela-

tion technique. Correlations among the test scores ranged from .80 to .98. Validity was based on the test's ability to differentiate children on their facility in using receptive language. Significant differences appeared in all age levels in the *Words* portions of the test as well as in total scores.

5. Additional Comments: It has been demonstrated that there is an interrelationship between proficiency in speechreading and proficiency in reading. It has also been demonstrated that ability to speechread and facets of mental ability are related.

6. Publisher: Grune and Stratton, Inc.
757 Third Avenue
New York, NY 10017

C. Goldman-Fristoe Test of Articulation

1. Purpose: Designed to assess an individual's articulation skills. Appropriate for ages 2 and over. Evaluates speechsound discrimination under both quiet and distracting noise conditions.

2. Description: A notebook kit consisting of colorful stimulus pictures. Three subtests include: (a) picture naming, (b) imitation of sounds in syllables, words, and sentences, and (c) story repetition. These subtests are provided in order to obtain a wide-range sample of a child's articulatory skills.

3. Administration: Is individually administered.

	The child is evaluated on three levels of complexity. Subject responds to a series of drawings by pointing to one of four pictures on a plate. Takes approximately 10 to 15 mintues to administer.
4. Technical Data:	Content validity has been adequately established. Reliability data reported appears to be satisfactory but incomplete. Only reported on two subtests. Standardized on 745 subjects from the general population at all age levels.
5. Additional Comments:	This test appears to have some promise as a tool used in the planning of speech therapy for all handicapped children.
6. Publisher:	American Guidance Service, Inc. Publishers Building Circle Pines, MN 55014

D. Test for Auditory Comprehension of Language

1. Purpose:	Can be adopted to assess language comprehension for the hearing impaired and the handicapped population. Appropriate for use with children ages 3 to 7 years.
2. Description:	Test consists of 101 pictures to which the child responds to an oral stimulus by pointing to one of three drawings.
3. Administration:	Individually administered. Takes approximately 20 minutes.
4. Technical Data:	Reliability established by test-retest method. Correlation coefficient of .94 was established by this procedure. Validity coefficient of .80 was established by

correlation of scores with IQs of mentally retarded children.

5. Additional Comments: Scores can be compared on an item-by-item basis with norm-referenced population. Mental age, syntax morphology, and vocabulary scores can be obtained.

6. Publisher: Learning Concepts
2501 N. Lamar
Austin, TX 78705

E. Verbal Language Development Scale

1. Purpose: Means of obtaining a measure of language development on those who are otherwise difficult to measure.

2. Description: The VLDS is an expansion of the verbal portion of the Vineland Social Maturity Scale. It yields a language age equivalent based on a child's level of communication. Appropriate for ages 1 month to 16 years.

3. Administration: The informant-interview method is used. Test is untimed.

4. Technical Data: Reliability is reported in terms of test-retest method. Correlations of .96 have been reported for both normal and retarded children using this procedure. Validity was determined by comparing VLDS scores with clinical ratings of language development utilizing the method. Correlations of .91 and .94 were respectively reported for normal and retarded subjects. The scale was standardized on a total of 237 children representative in respect to urban-rural res-

	idence, socioeconomic level, and sex.
5. Additional Comments:	The way in which the test is administered makes it possible to use for a number of different handicaps.
6. Publisher:	Educational Test Bureau
	Division of American Guidance Services, Inc.
	720 Washington Avenue, S.E.
	Minneapolis, MN 55414

ASSESSMENT GUIDELINES
Deaf and Hearing Impaired

III. Motor-Perceptual Development

A. Deaf-Blind Program and Ability Screening Test

   1. Purpose: Designed to determine the individual functioning and program needs of persons with multiple visual and auditory handicaps, Includes: gross and fine motor skills. Other pertinent data have been provided in previous sections (see page 126).

B. Marianne Frostig Developmental Test of Visual Perception

   1. Purpose: A test of visual perception which yields information regarding child's methods of processing information.

   2. Description: Five perceptual areas are included because of their reported relationship to early school performance. Appropriate for ages 3 to 8 years.

   3. Administration: May be administered individually or in small groups. May also be used with deaf or hard of hearing.

   4. Technical Data: Reliability is not high. Test-retest reliability of the perceptual quotient is reported to be .80 for a group of first and second graders, with subtest reliabilities ranging from .42 to .80. Results of validation studies indicate a lack of support for Frostig's definition of the figure-ground and form constancy subtests but support for the subtest position in

space. Also does not discriminate poor readers from good readers at the first grade level, with modest correlations of .40 to .50 being reported. Test-retest reliability for kindergarten and first graders ranges from .29 to .74.

5. Additional Comments: The Frostig DTVP does not appear to do a good job of assessing specific areas of perception differentially. Children from low socioeconomic groups and minority groups are poorly represented.

6. Publisher: Consulting Psychologists Press, Inc.
577 College Avenue
Palo Alto, CA 94306

C. Oseretsky Tests of Motor Proficiency

1. Purpose: An individual test of motor development for subjects 4 to 16 years.

2. Description: The Oseretsky Tests comprise a year-by-year scale of both fine and gross motor developments of children. Five basic types of tasks are included for each age: general static coordination, general dynamic coordination, motor speech, simultaneous voluntary movements, performance without extraneous movements.

3. Administration: Individually administered. Takes approximately 20 to 30 minutes. Pantomime demonstrations of the instructions reduce the intellectual component in performance and make it suitable for

	deaf and hard-of-hearing subjects.
4. Technical Data:	Not reported.
5. Additional Comments:	It appears that statistical study is needed before this test can be of any practical value.
6. Publisher:	American Guidance Services, Inc. Publisher's Building Circle Pines, MN 55014

D. Developmental Test of Visual-Motor Integration

1. Purpose:	To assess the degree to which visual perception and motor behavior are integrated. Designed for ages 2 to 15 years.
2. Description:	Consists of 24 geometric forms to be copied in a test booklet.
3. Administration:	Can be administered to groups as well as individual children. No time limit.
4. Technical Data:	Validity studies are somewhat mixed. A correlation of .89 between scores on the VMI and chronological age is reported. Other studies show that the correlation with mental age increases from .59 to .83 from the first to the seventh grade. Test-retest reliability over a two-week period for all age levels is as follows: boys .83, girls .87.
5. Additional Comments:	No differential information is reported by age group on reliability or validity. Test standardization appears to be adequate only for children ages 5 to 13 from suburban schools. For children below 5 years this test appears to be of limited use.

6. Publisher: Developmental Test
                         Follette Publishing Company
                         1010 West Washington Blvd.
                         Chicago, IL 60607

ASSESSMENT GUIDELINES
Deaf and Hearing Impaired

IV. Self-Help

A. Callier-Azusa Scale
   1. Purpose: To assess specific areas of development for deaf-blind and multi-handicapped children
   2. Description: This scale is comprised of 4 major areas including daily living skills. Within each area are 3 or 4 subscales made up of 6 to 17 developmentally sequential steps describing developmental milestones. Great detail is extended to the task analysis of such independent skills as toileting, dressing, and communcation, Goes up to 9 years of age.
   3. Administration: Individually administered. The observer or rater ascertains the highest specific step on each subscale which describes the developmental level of the child.
   4. Technical Data: Reliability was determined on the basis of correlations derived from inter-observer teams independently evaluating the child's behavior on each of the 16 subscales. These correlations ranged from .71 to .94.
   5. Additional Comments: A useful scale for planning developmentally appropriate programs for individual children. Although it can be administered by one person, most valid results are obtained if several individuals having close contact with

the child rate him on a consensus basis.

6. Publisher: Callier Center for Communication Disorders
1966 Inwood Road
Dallas, TX 75235

B. Camelot Behavioral Checklist
1. Purpose: To ascertain developmental level of individual, i.e. what the person can and cannot do.
2. Description: A behavioral checklist of 339 behavioral objectives arranged in age-expectancy order. Appropriate for all ages.
3. Administration: Individually administered. Takes approximately 15 to 30 minutes.
4. Technical Data: Reliability was reported by means of 2 independent teams evaluating 50 subjects. Correlation coefficients for various subtest ranged from .60 to .98 with a coefficient of .93 reported for the entire scale. Validity was established by correlating the Camelot with eight psychometric instruments that measure general intelligence. Correlations ranged from .33 to .86; all were significant at the .05 level or greater.
5. Additional Comments: The Camelot Behavioral Systems provides training programs and material packages in each area where the child is weak. Although designed for mentally retarded, it can be used with other handicapped populations.
6. Publisher: Camelot Behavioral Systems
P. O. Box 3447

Lawrence, KS 66044

C. Psychoeducational Inventory of Basic Skills and Personal
Development

    1. Purpose: A checklist designed to estimate a child's developmental level based upon observation of his behavior. Includes an area on self-care.

    2. Description: Behaviors included in the checklist are grouped into the following areas of functioning: social-emotional development, sensory discrimination, gross motor development, visual-motor coordination, perceptual integration, academic skills, and self-care. This inventory represents a method of organizing experience for children who could not organize and integrate their own.

    3. Administration: The inventory requires no special training to administer. It is individually administered by checking those items in which there is some observable evidence that the ability is present.

    4. Technical Data: This is not a standardized instrument. No technical data have been reported.

    5. Additional Comments: The inventory attempts to provide a convenient method of evaluating the child's development by categorizing discrete observable behaviors and arranging them in a normal sequence.

    6. Publisher: Mafex Associates, Inc.
90 Cherry Street
Johnstown, PA 15902

ASSESSMENT GUIDELINES
Deaf and Hearing Impaired

V. Social-Affective Behavior

A. Deaf-Blind Program and Ability Screening Test

   1. Purpose: To determine the individual's functioning of handicapped persons including the area of socialization. Other pertinent data have been described previously.

B. Devereux Child Behavior Rating Scale

   1. Purpose: To assess behavior of typical children ages 8 to 12.

   2. Description: Includes ratings on 17 different subparts of the scale including: distractibility, emotional detachment, social isolation, inadequate need for independence, social aggression, proneness to emotional upset, etc.

   3. Administration: The scale should be completed by one person who has general knowledge of the child's behavior.

   4. Technical Data: Reliability was determined by the test-retest method over a one-week time interval. A correlation coefficient of .83 was established by this procedure. Validity is not reported.

   5. Additional Comments: The Devereux appears to be moderately useful as a classification instrument used to provide treatment or for assessing behavioral changes.

   6. Publisher: The Devereux Foundation Press Devor, PA 19333

CHAPTER FIVE

ASSESSMENT GUIDELINES FOR THE VISUALLY IMPAIRED

ROBERT ROBINSON, PH.D.

VISUALLY IMPAIRED

$\mathbf{A}$ MAJOR concern in the selection of tests for the blind is undeniably related to such important questions as appropriateness and validity. In examining the current trends in test usage and the diagnostic problems unique to the blind, it is apparent that many test instruments have a predominant visual component and, as a result, are not usable with blind subjects. Similarly, almost all of the test instruments presently approved or recommended for use in the assessment of the blind have been based upon models designed for normally sighted populations. While the use of such instruments might be appropriate for some blind people, they might prove to be invalid for others.

Consequently, psychological testing with the blind appears to be, in many respects, a highly subjective clinical practice, the validity of which is difficult to gauge.

To assess the adequacy of test instruments as originally designed for a normally sighted population, or adapted for those who are blind, it is necessary to first consider the impact blindness has upon the total organization of the individual. Furthermore, we should always keep in mind that the term "the blind" is really a collection of subgroups of persons who have some visual impairment and that there are important behavioral differences between those who are congenitally blind and those who become blind later in life. There are also important behavioral differences among those with differing levels of vision. In brief, blindness affects each person in a unique way. A person never becomes fully adjusted to his loss of vision but, rather, constantly engages in a process of making more effective adjustments to it just as everyone, disabled or not, continually makes adjustments to a total life situation. In other words, it should be recognized that the types and degrees of adjustments made to blindness are conditioned by the person's total organization even before the loss of sight, and that two people, even with the same degree of measured visual acuity, often do not perceive in the same way.

In the creation of new test instruments for the blind, and in the adaptations of existing ones, testers have failed thus far to explore or question what vital differences, if any, accrue to learning and behavior as a result of being born blind or of losing sight later in life. For example, in the congenitally blind youngster we must question whether it is tenable to assume that even the words that are used in the formal testing situation have the same meaning as they might with sighted youngsters or children whose blindness occurred after language was established. Consider, for example, the vast differences in the coping or accommodating mechanisms used by blind infants during the sensorimotor stage of development (as compared to the sighted) and the impact of the early assimilation of knowledge on later perceptions and thought. In other words, the blind child first must experience his environment in his own unique way, then has to reorganize much of his assimilation to learn the way the sighted perceives this same environment. It must be recognized that this process of learning, unlearning, and relearning is extremely complicated for the congenitally blind and, as a result, affects accommodation and integration at each developmental stage. In effect, it can be hypothesized that the formation of intelligence in the congenitally blind may be different in important ways from that of the sighted, and that testing of the blind may require a uniquely different approach if we are to understand and assess a blind individual's intellectual potential.

Too frequently an evaluation or appraisal is automatically interpreted as prognosis instead of merely an assessment of the individual's characteristics at a given time and place under given circumstances. The confusion of diagnosis with prognosis tends to lead to a vicious cycle. When a person is regarded as unable to learn a certain task, he is excluded from certain training programs and thus deprived of the opportunity to prove himself. The subsequent poor performance is then regarded as bearing out the initial low estimation of his capacity.

In assessing blind children for the purpose of identifying potential for further education and training, it is very important not to accept ratings at face value. Instead, it is necessary to establish whether or not the child has had an opportunity to do those things expected of someone his age and whether or not, after he has been adequately stimulated, he is still unable to do such tasks. If a person's performance on a test is viewed as being influenced primarily by what he has learned, as opposed to innate capacity, then one is less likely to make long-run predictions about his ultimate success in school or a job on the basis of a test score.

The point that needs to be emphasized is that the diagnostic function, if it is to have any value, must be kept dynamic. Analysis and description of individuals must be done in functional behavioral terminology and not diagnostic labels. Too often the label or score summarized a complex interrelated pattern of many different facets of response. The uniqueness of the individual can only be understood in highlighting the uniqueness of his current pattern of responding. Only in this way can assistance be provided in planning for what can be done to help.

Finally, evaluation procedures should include an individual's appraisal of himself in the continuum of sighted-to-blind, especially since most blind persons see themselves as sighted and behave in accordance with this self-perception. In terms of test norms this implies that three distinct populations have to be considered: the congenitally blind, the partially sighted, and acquired or adventitious blindness.

REVIEW OF TEST INSTRUMENTS FOR THE BLIND AND VISUALLY IMPAIRED

The following section includes a review of various assessment instruments that are appropriate in testing the blind and visually impaired. These instruments have been categorized under the specific headings as follows: Intellectual Assessment, Language Skills, Motor-Perceptual, Development, Self-Help, and Social-Affective.

ASSESSMENT GUIDELINES
Blind and Visually Impaired

I. INTELLECTUAL ASSESSMENT

A. Haptic Intelligence Scale

1. Purpose: Nonverbal test used to measure the intelligence of blind adults.

2. Description: Consists of six subtests, four of which are modified adaptations of the performance scale of the WAIS.

3. Administration: Individually administered. Requires tactile discrimination and skillful manipulation of parts.

4. Technical Data: Test-retest reliability for the total test was .94. Reliability for individual subtests range from .70 to .81. Validity was determined by comparing performance of blind group (ages 20 to 34) with the WAIS verbal. A correlation of .65 was established.

5. Additional Comments: Test has limitations when used with partially sighted. Since it is based on a tactile approach, even slightest view of the materials invalidates the subject's performance. Also there is some question as to whether partially sighted persons develop the necessary tactile skill as do the blind. Test should be used in conjunction with other verbal tests of intelligence.

6. Publisher: Psychology Research
Box 14, Technology Center
Chicago, IL 60616

B. Raven Progressive Matrices for Presentation to the Blind (Tactual Progressive Matrices)

1. Purpose: An intellectual measure for the adult blind.

2. Description: 50 items — raised tactual designs on heavy illustration board. Task is to select correct pattern piece for completing the progress of the pattern in the matrix.

3. Administration: Individually administered. Takes approximately 40 minutes to administer.

4. Technical Data: A validity coefficient of .49 was established by correlating scores with the WAIS. A reliability coefficient of .95 was established by the split-half technique.

5. Additional Comments: Test standardized on 122 adult persons with vision poorer than 5/200 by Snellen index or equivalent of 99% loss of full visual acuity.

6. Publisher: Robert P. Anderson
Department of Psychology
Texas Tech University
Lubbock, TX 79410

C. Wechsler Intelligence Scale for Children revised and Wechsler Adult Intelligence Scale (Verbal Portions)

1. Purpose: As is true with other nonhandicapped individuals, these tests can provide a fairly good measure of verbal intelligence for blind subjects. However, it should be kept in mind that these instruments did not include any blind subjects in the standardization sample. Practical experience has shown that all of the performance items, with the exception of Picture Arrange-

ment, can be successfully utilized with visually impaired subjects whose vision is only 5/200. Furthermore, it has been found that most visually handicapped persons are able to complete these performance items within the normal time limits. On the other hand, it is important not to feel constricted by time limits as the basic intent of any evaluation is to determine how much the subject is capable of performing. If undue concern and attention are given to time limits in assessing certain handicapped persons such as the blind, then the testing is likely to result in a disservice to the client rather than being of benefit.

D. Kahn Intelligence Test
   1. Purpose: An intelligence scale that can be used with blind subjects. Other pertinent data have been presented previously (see page 117).

E. Perkins-Binet Test of Intelligence for the Blind
   1. Purpose: To evaluate the intelligence of the blind and visually impaired.
   2. Description: Consists of two forms: Form U, which is suitable for subjects with usable vision, and Form N, which is suitable for subjects with nonusable vision. Subtests on both forms consist of various items from the Binet. Items on Form N are primarily verbal in nature and go from age 4 to 18. Form U combines both performance and verbal items which

	extend from ages 3 to 17. Both forms cover a wide range of areas.
3. Administration:	Individually administered. Braille material is provided in all but a few subtests where oral testing is sufficient.
4. Technical Data:	The Perkins-Binet Test has been normed on a total sample of 2,146 children in schools from New England to California. From this sample, 49% were residential school students and 51% were day school students. Of the two forms, 828 students comprised the Form N or nonusable vision group, whereas the sample that was used for the usable vision group consisted of 1,318 students. No data for validity and reliability have been reported at this time.
5. Additional Comments:	The Perkins-Binet is not available on the market at this time but is expected to be sometime during the 1980-81 school year.
6. Publisher:	Perkins School for the Blind Watertown, MA 02172

F. The Blind Learning Aptitude Test

1. Purpose:	The BLAT is designed to provide a measure of the learning potential of blind persons for ages 6 to 20.
2. Description:	This test consists of a series of embossed items assessing the learning capabilities of blind students in generalization, discrimination, sequencing, analogies, and pattern or matrix completion.

3. Administration: Individually administered with no time limits. Performance on the items requires very little verbal response.

4. Technical Data: The BLAT was standardized on 961 blind subjects in residential schools of 12 states, which included 55 day schools in sixteen cities. Reliability was obtained by employing the Kuder-Richardson Formula. A correlation coefficient of .93 was established for the total age range. Validity was computed by correlating performance on the BLAT with Hayes-Binet and WISC verbal measures. This resulted in correlations of .74 with the Hayes-Binet and .71 with the WISC verbal.

5. Additional Comments: The BLAT predominantly processes those psychological operations which are necessary for learning. No fine tactual discrimination is called for in the solution of the test items nor is any reading of Braille.

6. Publisher: University of Illinois Press
Urbana, IL 61801

ASSESSMENT GUIDELINES
Blind and Visually Impaired

II. LANGUAGE SKILLS

A. Developmental Checklist
  1. Purpose:
Designed to assess the visually handicapped in the basic areas of child development including: receptive language and expressive language. Appropriate for ages 1 to 8.

  2. Description:
In addition to the language scale, this checklist covers other basic areas of child development such as self-help, social skills, gross and fine motor skills. Also included is an orientation and mobility section which is unique to the development of a visually handicapped child.

  3. Administration:
The Developmental Checklist may be administered either through direct observation or reliable reporting by a person familiar with the child. Space has been provided to administer the checklist up to four times a year, checking off those skills the child has mastered and leaving blank those he/she has not.

  4. Technical Data:
No attempt was made to develop technical data as the purpose was to design an instrument that had practical utility.

  5. Additional Comments: This checklist is specifically designed for use with children having varying degrees of visual impairment. Checklist method

		also allows for the recording of smaller increments of gain than multi-handicapped children typically make.
6.	Publisher:	Boston Center for Blind Children
		147 South Huntington Avenue
		Boston, MA 02130

ASSESSMENT GUIDELINES
Blind and Visually Impaired

III. MOTOR SKILL DEVELOPMENT

A. Deaf-Blind Program and Ability Screening Test
   1. Purpose: Designed to determine the individual functioning of handicapped persons in several areas, including: gross and fine motor skills. Other pertinent data have been presented previously (see page 126).

B. Developmental Checklist
   1. Purpose: Designed to assess the visually handicapped in 8 basic areas including: gross and fine motor skills. Other pertinent data have been presented previously (see page 148).

C. Psychoeducational Inventory of Basic Skills and Personal Development
   1. Purpose: A checklist designed to estimate a child's development in 7 basic areas including: gross motor and visual-motor integration. Other pertinent data have been presented previously (see page 138).

ASSESSMENT GUIDELINES
Blind and Visually Impaired

IV. SELF-HELP

A. Maxfield-Bucholz Scale of Social Maturity for Use With Preschool Blind Children

1. Purpose: To assess social competence of young blind children in 7 basic areas. Includes: self-help general, self-help dressing, and self-help eating.

2. Description: Scale covers age range of birth to 6 years. Consists of 95 items each placed within the year level of expected performance.

3. Administration: Scale is administered by an interview with an informant having intimate knowledge of the child. Evidence also gained from direct observation of the child. Each item scored in same way as Vineland Scale; i.e. +, − ,and ± (plus-minus).

4. Technical Data: The scale was normed on 484 children who were considered legally blind. No measures of reliability have been established as yet. Validity was established by the percent passing technique with most items following within the 80% range for children of the CA group.

5. Additional Comments: Some problems with respect to internal consistency. There are different numbers of items in the various categories, and the categories are unevenly represented throughout the scale.

6. Publisher: American Foundation for the Blind, Inc.
15 West 16th Street
New York, NY 10011

B. Callier-Azusa Scale
1. Purpose: A developmental scale designed for use with deaf-blind and multi-handicapped children. Scale is appropriate for ages birth through 9 years. Other pertinent data have been presented previously (see page 136).

C. Deaf-Blind Program and Ability Screening Test
1. Purpose: Assesses functioning in 7 developmental areas, including: self-help skills. Other pertinent data have been presented previously (see page 126).

D. Psychoeducational Inventory of Personal Development
1. Purpose: A checklist designed to estimate child's development in 7 areas of functioning, including: self-care. Other pertinent data have been presented previously (see page 138).

E. A Manual for the Assessment of a Deaf-Blind, Multiple Handicapped Child
1. Purpose: A comprehensive checklist designed to assess various levels of development for deaf-blind children. Suitable for early childhood age level.

2. Description: Instrument comprised of 6 developmental scales: personal self-help skills, social development, gross and fine motor development, communication, and cognition. Scales include comprehensive forms for background

	information, physical condition and developmental scales.
3. Administration:	Individually administered. Takes approximately 15 to 30 minutes.
4. Technical Data:	Instrument standardized on 350 deaf-blind children. No reliability and validity reported.
5. Additional Comments:	Scales can serve as a guide for training parents and para-professional aides.
6. Publisher:	Midwest Regional Resource Center for Service to Deaf-Blind Children
	P. O. Box 240
	Lansing, MI 48902

ASSESSMENT GUIDELINES
Blind and Visually Impaired

V. SOCIAL-AFFECTIVE BEHAVIOR

A. Deaf-Blind Program and Ability Screening Test
   1. Purpose: To assess functioning in 7 developmental areas, including: socialization. Other pertinent data have been described previously.

B. Maxfield-Bucholz Scale of Social Maturity for Use With Preschool Blind Children
   1. Purpose: To assess young blind children in 7 basic areas, including: socialization. Other pertinent data have been described previously.

C. Developmental Checklist
   1. Purpose: To assess blind children (ages 1 to 8) in 8 areas of child development, including: socialization. Other pertinent data have been presented previously.

CHAPTER SIX

ASSESSMENT GUIDELINES FOR THE PHYSICALLY HANDICAPPED

ROBERT ROBINSON, PH.D.

TESTING THE PHYSICALLY HANDICAPPED

THE motor, speech, visual, and auditory difficulties of physically handicapped children not only limit the applicability of standardized tests and testing procedures, but also make it necessary to exercise a good deal of caution in interpreting test results. On the other hand, standardized tests and techniques should be employed wherever possible because it is important to be able to determine what capacity the physically handicapped child has to adjust to the demands of life and to compete with those who are not handicapped.

Of the variety of general intelligence and educational tests, the psychologist needs to be able to select those instruments that suit the purpose for which the examination is given. Due to the fact that a comprehensive evaluation calls for a study of the total child rather than just intellectual functioning, the use of supplementary tests will be needed because they provide more opportunities for a greater variety and increased number of samples of behavior. In addition to exploring more areas of competencies, supplementary tests also enable the examiner to explore a particular area in-depth.

The actual administration of tests for the physically handicapped presents some rather serious problems. Because many of these children are disturbed by noises and are easily overstimulated by movements, objects, and bright colors, the merits of examining some children in their own homes should first be considered. Similarly, the very fearful or insecure child may respond most adequately in his familiar surroundings.

Test Modification Procedures

From the time testing is undertaken, the examiner must find appropriate ways of modifying existing test materials and/or procedures so as to allow the physically handicapped child to respond to test items. Some of the more flexible approaches in using standardized tests include: the elimination of time limits, using test items in a multiple choice situation though they were not standardized in this manner, and permitting a parent to interpret or repeat a child's response.

There are various other ways of developing controlled modification procedures to aid the child in the testing situation. For example, a useful approach for the child who cannot pick up flat objects because of a hand coordination problem is to screw small knobs in these objects so as to facilitate picking them up and placing them. This type of child may also have difficulty in counting out blocks or objects because of poor hand control rather than because of a weakness in understanding number concepts. If this is the case, it is possible to have colored squares or circles drawn in a row on a long piece of paper and have the child indicate by pointing to the place representing the specified number. Similarly, for the child who cannot manipulate small objects, such as stringing beads, it is possible to find out if the child remembers the pattern by having him place the beads in the correct order on a table.

The substitution of large objects for small ones and large pictures for small ones is also recommended in those cases where children have difficulty in either discerning or handling small objects. In a similar vein, problems are generally encountered with children who do not have enough hand control to complete drawings either as a response to verbal directions or in copying from a presented pattern. Consequently, the suitability of such tests has been questioned. Though some children cannot move a hand, many others with severe limitations in the use of hands are able to draw well enough to enable the examiner to differentiate between a lack of understanding and an inability to coordinate well enough to produce a form accurately. If the child is carefully observed while drawing, it is possible in many instances to make this differentiation.

The evaluation or scoring of a drawing is also subject to many errors if it is done without observation of the child as he draws.

Object assembly and block design tests perhaps offer the greatest complications when there is hand involvement. However, if the problems associated with these tests can be overcome, it is desirable to utilize them as they can supply specific clues to problems in perception and organization that may be associated with neurological dysfunctioning. There are several useful procedures that can be used to assist those subjects who, in placing blocks or other parts of a test, unavoidably move all other pieces, thus disrupting the pattern. The examiner may help by holding the pieces firmly, thus enabling the subject to continue. However, care must be exercised to make no change in the position of any piece except at the request of the subject. In working with block designs, it will be helpful to use frames in which the finished pattern will fit. The construction of a frame will eliminate the necessity of lifting the blocks as they can be pushed into place. Prior to the use of such a device, it must be known that the subject is able to visualize the finished design as a square. It must also be used in such a way as to give no clues to the solution of the problem.

There are other modifications or adaptations that can be worked out in making use of nonverbal or performance tests. For example, a picture arrangement test, usually made of thin material, is very difficult to handle. Mounting the original pictures on heavy cardboard may thus make it possible for many subjects with hand involvement to arrange them. If it is too difficult in spite of the adaptation, the subject may merely indicate the card he wants in each position and the examiner can place it.

For the child who has verbal comprehension but cannot talk, many verbal questions can be answered by a yes or no shake of the head. Picture completion tests can also be administered to subjects who lack speech by having them point to the missing part of the pictures or the corresponding parts of themselves or to objects in the room if they are applicable. In an effort to gain some understanding of the nontalking child's level of attainment in the areas of letter and number recognition, simple number work, and in spelling, it is possible to have the child knock down large plastic numbers and letters that he wants to designate. With regard to repeating digits, nontalking children may either write the series or in some instances point to the correct numbers after the printed numbers have been arranged in a one-to-ten order.

As was previously indicated, time limits must be frequently ignored with physically handicapped children. For example, in a performance type of test, it may be apparent that the child knows how to arrange the material but is physically unable to manipulate it within the given time. Giving the child unlimited time yields useful information in that it is possible for the examiner to observe the child's approach to problem solving, to discern the child's degree of understanding, and to note the actual level of accomplishment. By the same token, eliminating time limits with such tasks also enables the examiner to evaluate the qualitative factors involved in this type of test item. For instance, in naming words, a task found at the ten-year age level in the Stanford Binet Test, it may be valuable to know if there are long lapses in which the subject cannot think of any word; if he can name only words in a single category; or if he may be limited to associations by sound. This procedure may also give some indication of the range of the child's thinking and, together with other data, show if there is a certain range of practical interests, with corresponding ability to deal with the abstract.

Despite how much the psychologist tries to adapt tests or procedures to accommodate the child's handicaps, it will still be necessary to eliminate some tests. It is, however, necessary to distinguish between those tests that are impossible for the child because of physical involvement and those which are beyond his level of comprehension. In general, it has been found that it is easier to overestimate a child's ability than to underestimate it. Similarly, it is frequently an easy matter to stretch a point in the child's favor.

Some children are easily fatigued or frustrated when failures begin to pile up and cease to make further efforts. Hence, it is necessary to be keenly aware of the child's emotional reactions during the testing in order to handle the problem at the time it occurs. The practice of using subtests in an irregular order is an effective measure that frequently seems to help the small child who has difficulty in shifting his mental set quickly. For example, some small children tend to perseverate, which is not necessarily an outcome of poverty of thought. If a test is discontinued at the point that this occurs and resumed later, the child may be more likely to provide the correct response. This practice of spacing tasks where there is an element of sameness or repetitiveness can be very helpful in that it makes it possible to differentiate between a pattern that may well be an aspect of brain damage and a lack of the necessary mental ability to handle the task.

In summary, the recommended procedure for both handicapped children and adults is to let individuals complete tests in the standard manner if they can; if there must be modifications of tests or procedures, devise ways to learn how much the subject understands. If he cannot do it all, eliminate what is necessary and let the individual do what he can. Give full credit when earned, and promote when indicated. Form an estimate and acknowledge that it is an estimate, when that is the best that can be done.

Evaluating Test Results

Since it has been suggested that modifications in test items and/or procedures may invalidate the norms that have been established on a nonhandicapped population, the question has been raised by some as to why use standardized tests at all. First, it should be recognized that this is the only way of applying tests at all to many physically handicapped children. Second, this practice gives more accurate information than could possibly be secured by eliminating all those tests where the child cannot cooperate fully because of physical disabilities. Third, regardless of how imprecise the measure, no testing is valid if we cannot, to some extent, approximate how the physically handicapped child compares in performance with the nonhandicapped child.

In evaluating the significance of the results of a test that may have been administered in an unorthodox manner and standardized on normal children, it must be recognized that a great deal of clinical judgment enters into the evaluation and that many observations have probably contributed to the conclusions. Similarly, parents' descriptions of the child's reactions and experiences in the home may play an essential part in contributing to a more complete understanding and evaluation of the child.

In general, test results need to be evaluated in two ways: one must evaluate the child's current level of functioning and his probable potential. One way of doing this is to examine the range of the handicapped child's success in a given area or on a particular test. The highest level at which he is capable of functioning may represent his potential, especially if there is some consistency noted, and the lower levels represent his present level of functioning.

Finally, a statement as to how well the test represents the child should be included in every evaluation. Similarly, there should be no objection in admitting that the conclusions are tentative, if this proves to be the case, or in expressing a need of modifying results as further information dictates.

REVIEW OF TEST INSTRUMENTS FOR THE PHYSICALLY HANDICAPPED

The following section includes a review of various assessment instruments that are appropriate in testing the physically handicapped. These instruments have been categorized under the specific headings as follows: Intellectual Assessment, Language Skills, Motor-Perceptual Development, Self-Help, and Social-Affective.

ASSESSMENT GUIDELINES
Physically Handicapped

I. INTELLECTUAL ASSESSMENT

A. Quick Test

1. Purpose:	To provide a means of quick screening an individual's verbal intelligence in practical situations. Useful for assessing the mentality of the physically handicapped for whom standard measures cannot be used.
2. Description:	Test consists of 50 words associated with appropriate pictures that best fit the word. Suitable for ages 2 and over.
3. Administration:	Individually administered. Subject is required to say for each word which of four pictures "best fits it."
4. Technical Data:	Reliability is reported in terms of interform coefficients and range from .60 to .96. Validity data consist chiefly of comparisons with the Full Range Picture to .93. Mental age norms are based on sample of 458 white children and adults.
5. Additional Comments:	Some of the pictures appear to be ambiguous or crude. Norms based on a relatively small sample size. Should be kept in mind that results represent an estimate of ability and should be supplemented with other test data.
6. Publisher:	Psychological Test Specialists Box 1441 Missoula, MT 59801

B. Pictorial Test of Intelligence

1. Purpose:	A measure of individual's verbal intelligence. Covers age range from 3 to 8 years.
2. Description:	Consists of 6 subtests arranged in order of difficulty: picture vocabulary, form discrimination, information and comprehension, similarities, size and number, and immediate recall.
3. Administration:	Individually administered, non-timed. Test requires only sufficient command of English to understand simple instructions. Responses to questions usually take the form of pointing to one of four pictures on test card. Drawings are spatially arranged so as to accommodate children who have motor problems of the hands or arms. The examiner can observe easily the eye movements of the child who has been instructed to just look at his answer.
4. Technical Data:	Standardization based on 1,830 children. Reliability reported in terms of test-retest reliability ranging from .90 to .96 for time intervals of two to six weeks. Validity is reported in terms of correlation between PTI and WISC and Binet scores of kindergarten children. Correlations of .75 and .78 respectively were obtained.
5. Additional Comments:	Although needing additional research, this test appears to have promise as an individual learn-

ing aptitude test for young children.

6. Publisher:
Houghton Mifflin Company
110 Fremont Street
Boston, MA 02107

C. Columbia Mental Maturity Scale
1. Purpose:
Designed to measure intelligence of handicapped children from 3 1/2 to 9 years 11 months of age.

2. Description:
A 100 item pictorial type classification test that utilizes perceptive discriminations involving color, shape, size, use, number, kind, missing parts, and symbolic materials.

3. Administration:
Individual administration with no time limit.

4. Technical Data:
Revised scale (1972) was standardized on a nonhandicapped population sample. A median test-retest reliability coefficient of .85 was obtained for three different age groups, 0-4 years through 5-8 years of age. Validity was established by obtaining correlations between the 1972 CMMS and the 1959 CMMS, the Otis-Lennon Mental Ability Test-Level I, and the Stanford Binet, Form L-M. The respective correlations obtained were .84, .63, and .67.

5. Additional Comments: Examiner should exercise caution in using results below the 4-year level. It has been reported that younger deaf children have difficulty comprehending what the examiner wants when he asks them to indicate the one

that does not belong. Also, perseveration may be encouraged at the lower levels by the fact that the correct answer tends to appear on the same number consecutively. Would recommend this test be used with a good bit of caution as information that is obtained may be of little practical use.

6. Publisher: Harcourt Brace and World, Inc.
757 Third Avenue
New York, NY 10017

D. Full-Range Picture Vocabulary Test

1. Purpose: To provide a measure of intelligence for special groups such as physically handicapped or persons with speech handicaps for whom standard measures cannot be used.

2. Description: Test is based on pictures which measure approximately the same factor or factors which underlie the Wechsler and Binet vocabulary tests. Consists of 16 plates each with four separate cartoon-like drawings on it. The testee is asked to indicate by word or gesture which of the pictures best illustrates the meaning of a given word. Approximately 80 words are used in each of two parallel forms which cover the range of verbal abilities from early infancy to the superior adult level.

3. Administration: Individually administered. Takes approximately 15 minutes or less.

4. Technical Data: Reliability is reported in comparing forms A and B on adult samples. A correlation of .93 was established by this means. Validity was established by comparing forms A and B with Stanford-Binet vocabulary raw scores. Correlations of .91 and .93 respectively were established by this procedure. The standardization sample included 80 Spanish-American and 80 Black children.

5. Additional Comments: Tests appears to have good validity as a quick verbal intelligence screening device in testing persons seriously handicapped by a speech defect or by upper extremity disabilities.

6. Publisher: Psychological Test Specialist
Box 1441
Missoula, MT 59801

E. Children's Picture Information Test

1. Purpose: To assess intelligence of children 2 to 6 years of age with motor handicaps or lacking oral skills.

2. Description: Test consists of 40 sets of colored pictures of which 4 alternatives goes with the picture. An effort was made to restrict the content largely to everyday household situations with which an immobilized child of confined environment would be familiar.

3. Administration: Individually administered. The child indicates by pointing or responding in some other discriminable way, which of 4 alternatives goes with the picture.

4. Technical Data: Standardized on 400 normal children aged 2 to 6 years in Seattle, Washington. In addition, 59 handicapped children included in sample. A test-retest reliability correlation coefficient of .93 was reported. Validity is reported in terms of product moment correlations of CPIT scores and Binet mental ages for normal and handicapped groups. Correlation coefficients of .89 and .80 respectively were obtained.

5. Additional Comments: Pictures are cut from children's books rather than designed to standard specifications. Hence, pictures differ in hue, clarity, scale relationships and fineness of detail.

6. Publisher: Spastic Aid Council, Inc.
1850 Boyer Avenue
Seattle, WA 98102

F. Peabody Picture Vocabulary Test
1. Purpose: To provide an estimate of individual's verbal intelligence. With modifications in administration instructions, can be used with physically handicapped by having individual nod head when presented with choices. Other pertinent data have been presented previously.

ASSESSMENT GUIDELINES
Physically Handicapped

II. LANGUAGE SKILLS

A. Reynell Developmental Language Scales
   1. Purpose: For the assessment of expressive language and verbal comprehension in handicapped children.
   2. Description: Appropriate for children ages 1 to 6. Expressive language scale contains 4 scores: language structure, vocabulary, content, and total. Contains a graph for girls and boys.
   3. Administration: Individually administered. Takes approximately 30 minutes to administer. Props are needed to administer test.
   4. Technical Data: The standardization sample consisted of not less than 50 children at each half year level from six months to six years inclusive. The exact number of the sample was 636 children. The geographical area covered was a wide area of London and the Southeast of England. Reliability coefficients were calculated for each age group in each scale using a split-half technique. Coefficients ranged from .77 to .92 respectively. No validity is reported at this time.
   5. Additional Comments: This experimental edition is intended to be used as a clinical tool for the use with handicapped children. This instrument has been developed over a period of 5 years.

6. Publisher: N.F.E.R. Publishing Company, Ltd.
                         2 Jennings Buildings, Thames Avenue
                         Windsor Berks, England

B. Utah Test of Language Development
  1. Purpose: Measures expressive and receptive verbal language skills in both normal and handicapped children. Can be administered to aphasic and brain-damaged individuals.
  2. Description: A 51 item instrument for measuring the expressive and receptive language skills of children ages 1 1/2 to 14 1/2. Items are equally divided between those which measure selective and those which measure sequential language facility. Includes a number of sequencing tasks such as repeating digits, repeating sentences, and indicating the days of the week.
  3. Administration: Individually administered. Test is untimed. Scoring sheet is simple and easy to use.
  4. Technical Data: Test standardized on 273 white, normal children in Utah. Reliability was determined by split-half correlation and is reported to be .94. Test items have face validity because they were selected from previously standardized sources.
  5. Additional Comments: The UTLD can be useful as a language screening device if supplemented with other tests. Children with visual-perceptual

problems, children from inner-city populations, and nonwhite children should be evaluated by other means. Can be a useful instrument at preschool level due to preponderance of items at this level.

6. Publisher: Communication Research Associates, Inc.
Box 11012
Salt Lake City, UT 84111

C. Verbal Language Development Scale

1. Purpose: A behavior checklist for use in interviewing adult informants regarding a child's performance on verbal tasks. Appropriate for use with children between ages of birth to 15.

2. Description: A 50 item scale which is an extension of the communication section of the Vineland Social Maturity Scale. These 50 items serve as a basis for obtaining language age equivalents as observed and evaluated by an adult.

3. Administration: Directions are brief, indicating examiner should elicit a response from the informant in such a way that responses are not biased. Informant's responses are to be scored plus, plus-minus, or minus after ascertaining whether the item is habitually performed, in an emergent state only, or "cursory" or absent.

4. Technical Data: Standardized on 120 normal speaking white children from central Utah. No substantial information is provided on validity

       and reliability studies.

5. Additional Comments: Use of the scale for inner-city, large urban centers or nonwhite children does not seem to be appropriate. Language ages achieved by the interview method are frequently much higher than those achieved by a language examination.

6. Publisher: American Guidance Service, Inc. Publishers Building Circle Pines, MN 55014

D. TARC Assessment Inventory for Severely Handicapped Children

1. Purpose: Provides a behavioral assessment of the capabilities of severe handicapped children on a number of skills including: communication.

2. Description: Yields scores in following areas: self-help motor, communication and social skills. Designed to assess young children ages 3 to 16.

3. Administration: Can be administered by parent or teacher. Scores are expressed in terms of standard scores by grade or developmental level. Takes approximately 15 to 30 minutes to administer.

4. Technical Data: Reliability is reported in terms of test-retest, which proved to be .80. Validity is not reported.

5. Additional Comments: Child should be observed a minimum of 13 weeks in a group or close setting before proceeding with testing.

6. Publisher: H and H Enterprises, Inc. P. O. Box 3342 Lawrence, KS 66044

E. Language and Learning Disorders of the Preacademic Child

    1. Purpose: Test is designed to provide information in helping to diagnose and remediate language and learning problems for children with various handicaps. Suitable for ages birth to 6 years.

    2. Description: Instrument is comprised of subtests in the areas of: comprehension of single words and connected discourse; expression of connected discourse; short-term auditory memory for digits and sentences; short-term visual memory for — paper folding, draw a man, and perceptual motor.

    3. Administration: Individually administered. Takes approximately 60 to 90 minutes to administer. Expresses scores by developmental level and mental age.

    4. Technical Data: None available.

    5. Additional Comments: This battery also attempts to identify the etiology as well as providing the means to demonstrate measured gains by reassessment.

    6. Publisher: Western Psychological Services
12031 Wilshire Boulevard
Los Angeles, CA 90025

F. Dailey Language Facility Test

    1. Purpose: Test is designed to assess the ability of persons with language problems to use oral language independently of vocabulary, information, pronunciation, and grammar.

2. Description: Test consists of a series of pictures that the subject describes or tells a story about. Suitable for subjects ages 3 to 18.

3. Administration: Individually administered. Responses to each picture are scored on a 9-point scale according to detailed criteria.

4. Technical Data: Reliability is reported in terms of the test-retest method ranging from .70 to .90. Test standardized on 4,000 Head Start Children throughout country and 1,700 persons, third grade through adulthood.

5. Additional Comments: Two scoring systems are provided. System I measures the child's ability to communicate in his own way, independent of standard English or grammatical exactness. The second system codes the errors or deviations from standard usage and provides a diagnostic profile of the child's ability to speak standard English.

6. Publisher: The Allington Corporation
801 North Pitt Street
Alexandria, VA 22314

G. Carrow Elicited Language Inventory
1. Purpose: An inventory that can be used to identify children with language problems. Designed for use with handicapped and early childhood children ages 3 to 8 years.

2. Description: A training guide and training tape accompany the material and can be used in follow-up practice for the child.

3. Administration: Individually administered. Testing time is approximately 45 minutes. Scores are expressed by percentiles and stanines.

4. Technical Data: Author reports correlation coefficients that range from .98 to .99. Concurrent validity is reported as .62.

5. Additional Comments: This inventory can also be used to determine the linguistic structure that contributes to the child's language problems.

6. Publisher: Learning Concepts
                            2501 N. Lamar
                            Austin, TX 78705

H. Environmental Language Inventory

1. Purpose: Test is designed to assess the preschool and severely handicapped child's language development. Suitable for children ages 2 to 6 years.

2. Description: The test assesses the child's sentence types in play, conversation, and limitation. Language development is measured by mean length of utterances.

3. Administration: Individually administered. Takes approximately 20 to 30 minutes. The content of the linguistic and nonlinguistic areas may be altered to suit the individual child.

4. Technical Data: No statistical data is reported. Test standardized on over 300 children seen at Nisonger Center.

5. Additional Comments: Parents can be used as aides in the language intervention program.

6. Publisher: Nisonger Center
Ohio State University
1580 Cannon Drive
Columbus, OH 43210

I. Bzoch-League Receptive-Expressive Emergent Language Scale: For the Measurement of Language in Infancy

1. Purpose: A test that can be used to measure expressive and receptive language with handicapped children — especially with the developmentally disabled.

2. Description: Test consists of 132 items of a behavioral nature. Includes 3 subtests: expressive language, receptive language, and combined language. Suitable for children from birth to 36 months.

3. Administration: Individually administered. Takes from 10 to 15 minutes and requires no speech by the child. Parent, nurse, or teacher can be used as respondent.

4. Technical Data: A reliability coefficient of .91 is reported. No validity scores are reported but author states that test correlates vary highly with the Verbal Standard Language Test. All racial-cultural groups were sampled in the standardization population.

5. Additional Comments: Test is widely used by physicians and provides a developmental score computed by a ratio formula.

6. Publisher: Anhinga Press
550 Park Avenue, East
Tallahassee, FL 32307

ASSESSMENT GUIDELINES
Physically Handicapped

III. MOTOR SKILL DEVELOPMENT

A. Behavioral Developmental Profile

1. Purpose: Designed to monitor development and profile an organized approach to skill acquisition.

2. Description: Intended for use with handicapped children. Assesses 3 categories of skills: Communication, Motor, and Social. Appropriate for use with ages birth to 6 years.

3. Administration: Administered by individual evaluator. Evaluation in each of the various categories should start with tasks the child can successfully do. Evaluation then proceeds until the child experiences failure for two consecutive age segments. The score sheet reflects a success level, an emergent skill area, and a cluster of skills the child cannot yet master. Each profile item is cross-referenced to behavioral objectives. The objectives reduce behaviors into sequential steps with strategies for implementing each objective.

4. Technical Data: Test items were based on patterns of "normal" child development. No other technical data were reported.

5. Additional Comments: The profile permits a systematic observation of a variety of skills. Can be used with a variety of handicapped populations. It is designed to facilitate individual-

ized prescriptive teaching of pre-school children within the home setting.

6. Publisher: Department of Special Education
Area Agency 6
9 Westwood Drive
Marshalltown, IA 50158

B. Deaf-Blind Programs and Ability Screening Test

1. Purpose: Designed to determine individual functioning and program needs of multiple handicapped persons in 7 developmental areas, including: gross motor skills and fine motor skills. Other pertinent data have been presented previously.

C. Preschool Attainment Record

1. Purpose: Designed to measure the physical, social, mental, and language attainments of children from 6 months to 7 years.

2. Description: The test is divided into eight areas with 14 age items in each category. Among the 8 areas are included: ambulation and manipulation. Scale is intended to be used to determine the developmental level of children for whom verbal intelligence tests are not appropriate. It is well adapted for testing aphasic children and children with cerebral palsy.

3. Administration: Items are scored $+, -$, or $\pm$ for pass, fail, and doubtful, respectively. Scoring determined on basis of an adult's report of the child's behavior in each area.

4. Technical Data: No normative data are presented. No reliability or validity information is reported.

5. Additional Comments: Despite lack of normative data, the PAR appears to be a good basic inventory of the behaviors of infants and young children based on maturation and social expectations in American culture.

6. Publisher: American Guidance Services, Inc.

Publishers Building
Circle Pines, MN 55014

D. Motor-Free Visual Perception Test

1. Purpose: A test designed to measure visual perceptual-motor development of nonverbal and motorically involved children. Appropriate for children ages 5 to 8 years.

2. Description: Test consists of 36 items and is divided into the following subtests: visual discrimination, figure-ground, spatial relations, visual closure, and visual memory.

3. Administration: Individually administered. Takes approximately 10 minutes.

4. Technical Data: Reliability established by the test-retest method. Coefficients of .77 to .83 were reported. Validity was reported in terms of construct validity and ranged from .31 to .73.

5. Additional Comments: Standardization population consisted of all races and SES levels from 22 states. Mode of responding to this test is by pointing.

6. Publisher: Academic Therapy Publications
1539 Fourth Street
San Rafael, CA 94901

E. Early Intervention Developmental Profile and Developmental Screening of Handicapped Infants

1. Purpose: A profile designed to supplement the diagnostic data provided by standardized testing instruments. The profile aids examiners in describing the child's present accomplishments in all areas of development.

2. Description: A comprehensive screening instrument containing six developmental sequences which normally emerge between birth and 36 months of age. Major milestones in the areas of language, gross motor, fine motor, social/emotional, self-care, and cognitive development are presented in 3-month intervals which reflect normal developmental patterns attained in the first 3 years of life.

3. Administration: Individually administered. Takes approximately 45 minutes. Each profile can be used 4 times to allow the evaluators and parents to see the child's progress from one evaluation to the next. The profile should be administered every 3 to 4 months.

4. Technical Data: Profile has not been validated on normal or handicapped children. It should, therefore, be used as a supplement rather than a replacement for formal evaluation.

5. Additional Comments: The profile allows educators to

develop a knowledge of each individual child's developmental patterns and rates over a period of time. This information can also be used to develop objectives and activities which are developmentally appropriate for each child's functional level.

6. Publisher: University of Michigan
Publication Distribution Service
615 East University
Ann Arbor, MI 48109

F. Learning Accomplishment Profile (LAP-D) Diagnostic Edition

1. Purpose: A developmental checklist designed for use with children who may be experiencing developmental delays. Suitable for children ages 0 to 6 years.

2. Description: An informal checklist designed to evaluate progress in areas of language, cognition, self-help, gross and fine motor skills.

3. Administration: Individually administered. Testing time takes about an hour.

4. Technical Data: Reliability has been established by means of inter-raters. Reliability coefficients of various subtests range from .68 to .94. Validity data is presently being collected.

5. Additional Comments: Test should only be used as a pretest/posttest until validity data has been collected and reported.

6. Publisher: Kaplan School Supply
600 Jonestown Road
Winston-Salem, NC 27103

ASSESSMENT GUIDELINES
Physically Handicapped

IV. SELF-HELP

A. Life-Space Survey
    1. Purpose: Designed to serve as an additional instrument to help determine the degree of capability or quality of experiences the child might be exposed to in his home, neighborhood, and community environment.

    2. Description: Child indicates by drawing lines on a map of all the places he goes by himself. Points out the areas in which the parents need to enrich the child's environmental experiences. Appropriate for ages 6 and up.

    3. Administration: No time limit. Can be administered individually or in small groups. May also be filled out by a parent.

    4. Technical Data: No norms have been established.

    5. Additional Comments: Can be useful as an aid in developing educational objectives as well as finding out some of the child's personal problems and needs.

    6. Publisher: Academic Therapy Publications
                      1539 Fourth Street
                      P. O. Box 899
                      San Rafael, CA 94901

B. A Manual for the Assessment of a Deaf-Blind Multiple Handicapped Child.
    1. Purpose: A comprehensive checklist designed to assess various levels of development for deaf-blind

children. Suitable for early childhood age level. Other pertinent data have been presented previously.

C. Meeting Street School Screening Test

1. Purpose: For children who experience developmental delays in visual-perceptual, motor control, and language skill areas.

2. Description: Instrument consists of motor patterning, visual perceptual-motor, and language subtest scales. Appropriate for children ages 5 to 7 1/2 years.

3. Administration: Individually administered. Takes approximately 15 to 20 minutes to administer.

4. Technical Data: Reliability was established by the test-retest and inter-raters methods. Reliability coefficients of .85 and .95 respectively were reported by these procedures. Validity was established by correlating this instrument with the ITPA and Frostig. Correlation coefficients of .77 and .57 were derived by this procedure.

5. Additional Comments: Test is designed for use by teachers, psychologists, and physicians.

6. Publisher: Crippled Children and Adults of Rhode Island, Inc.
667 Waterman Avenue
East Providence, RI 02914

D. Portage Project

1. Purpose: A checklist designed to assess a child's behavior in a number of developmental areas. Appropriate for all handicapped chil-

	dren ages birth to 5 years.
2. Description:	Consists of the following sub-tests: cognitive, self-help, motor, language, and socialization.
3. Administration:	Is to be administered in the home with parents serving as teachers.
4. Technical Data:	Test standardized on a population that included a variety of handicapping conditions. No validity or reliability has been reported by the authors.
5. Additional Comments:	Purpose of instrument is to help plan realistic goals that lead to additional skills. Each skill in test has been task analyzed and is referenced to a file card which describes how to teach that skill.
6. Publisher:	Comparative Educational Service Agency No. 12 Portage, WI 53901

ASSESSMENT GUIDELINES
Physically Handicapped

V. SOCIALIZATION

A. Parent Interview Form
  1. Purpose: Designed to obtain information from parents of orthopedically handicapped children in a number of areas, including: socialization.
B. Behavioral Developmental Profile
  1. Purpose: Designed for use with handicapped children in obtaining information in 3 basic areas, including: communication, motor and social. Appropriate for children ages birth to 6 years. Other pertinent data have been presented previously (see page 175).
C. TARC Assessment Inventory for Severely Handicapped Children
  1. Purpose: Provide a behavioral assessment of the capabilities of handicapped children on a number of skills, including: social skills. Other pertinent data have been presented previously (see page 170).

CHAPTER SEVEN

ASSESSMENT GUIDELINES FOR THE SEVERE AND MULTI-HANDICAPPED

Robert Robinson, Ph.D.

IN assessing children with different combinations of physical handicaps, the severity of the handicapping conditions as well as the number of handicaps will often militate against the examiner being able to obtain formal test data. The utilization of standardized tests with handicapped children is also limited by the following three difficulties: (1) They may not provide reliable differentiations in the range of the group scores; (2) The predictive validity for handicapped populations may be different from that for the standardization and validation groups, and (3) The validity of their interpretations is strongly dependent upon the opportunity and experiences handicapped children have had to learn the answers to the questions asked.

Consequently, the examiner will, by necessity, have to rely more on informal procedures such as observations, rating scales, simple checklists, parent interviews, and criterion-referenced tests. It has been found that behavioral data collected by these means provide not only the same information as standardized tests, but have the added advantage of not requiring the services of a trained psychologist (MacTurk and Neisworth 1978). Further, criterion-referenced measures are program specific, i.e. they can be tied directly to the program objectives developed for a given child.

In the final analysis, all assessment and diagnostic information should serve the same purpose, i.e. appropriate educational programming for all children. Edgar and Musch (1976) indicate that the assessment data most beneficial to teachers are those related to actual child behavior in critical developmental tasks. By using established lists of sequenced developmental behaviors, the teachers can pinpoint those skills a child can perform in given areas of development and those skills which should be taught next.

Cromwell et al. (1975) also stress the importance of the outcome of assessment activities as being the most important criterion for judging the quality and worth of assessment. In brief, if effective interventions result from assessment, then these activities will generally be judged as beneficial for the individual. Assessment that leads to or is followed by ineffective interventions will, by definition, be regarded as inadequate and of little benefit.

The focus on an outcome criterion in assessment thus implies a number of important concepts. First, prior to making a diagnosis and concomitant placement decision, there must be interventions available which are directly related to the diagnosis. Second, diagnoses are of value to the individual only if the information that is provided about treatment is related to diagnosis and if data exists to support the effectiveness of the treatment program. Third, since progress cannot be evaluated on the basis of one set of test data, assessment must be an ongoing process. Because assessment data are used primarily by teachers and need to be collected frequently over a period of time, teachers need to be directly involved in the assessment and collection of that data. Also, because teachers are the only professionals who can observe children in an educational setting over a period of time, this unique position makes them the most logical persons to conduct the ongoing assessment. It is therefore imperative that teachers be trained to be effective and efficient in assessing their students and have access to informal assessment tools and devices which enable them to collect data in their classrooms easily and with minimal interruption.

REVIEW OF TEST INSTRUMENTS FOR THE SEVERE AND MULTI-HANDICAPPED

The following section includes a review of various commercially produced instruments that can be easily and conveniently administered to collect data on severe and multi-handicapped children. Further, these instruments require no specialized training or licensing to administer and enable teachers and others to pinpoint more precisely childrens' skill levels so that appropriate intervention can be devised.

ASSESSMENT GUIDELINES
Severe and Multi-Handicapped

A. AAMD Adaptive Behavior Scales

   1. Purpose: A scale devised to provide an assessment for the mentally handicapped, emotionally maladjusted, or developmentally impaired individual. Information is provided on the individual's effectiveness in coping with his environment.

   2. Description: This test provides information on adaptive behavior functioning in 12 essential categories of daily living. The scale also provides a behavioral description of the individual assessed.

   3. Administration: The scale can be administered by people without a great deal of special training, as well as by professionals. The test requires approximately 20 to 30 minutes to administer.

   4. Technical Data: The assessment is a standardized test intended to describe the individual's daily functioning rather than compare his performance with the average performance of other individuals.

   5. Additional Comments: Because the assessment consists of a recording of behavioral observations, the test can be applied for all ages of individuals diagnosed as developmentally impaired.

   6. Publisher: American Association on Mental Deficiency
5201 Connecticut Avenue, N.W.
Washington, D.C. 20015

B. Allied Agencies Functional Profile: Developmental Training Program

1. Purpose:	The functional profile is a checklist of developmental skills and social traits that normal infants and young children usually acquire or can perform at certain ages. By completing the checklist, one can determine the approximate level of functioning for the child in each of six areas.
2. Description:	This profile assesses functioning in the following areas: social, cognitive, gross motor, fine motor, eating, and toileting.
3. Administration:	Can be administered by any person with basic knowledge and experience with normal growth and development of infants and young children.
4. Technical Data:	Not standardized.
5. Additional Comments:	This is a profile for normal, not handicapped children, but will give the assessor an idea of how a handicapped child compares to a normal child. It is also a gross indicator of functioning; no fine discrimination is made between levels.
6. Publisher:	Peoria Association for Retarded Citizens and United Cerebral Palsy of Peoria 320 E. Armstrong Avenue Peoria, IL 61603

C. Balthazar Scales of Adaptive Behavior

1. Purpose:	This scale is appropriate for assessing ambulatory severely/profoundly retarded individuals ages 5 to 57.

2. Description: The Balthazar Scale is comprised of two sections: scales of functional independence and 8 additional social scale categories describing coping behaviors.

3. Administration: Can be administered by teachers or aides through direct observation.

4. Technical Data: This instrument was standardized on residents of the Central Wisconsin Colony and Training School.

5. Additional Comments: This scale is recommended for providing objectives for the design and development of behavioral programs, for providing a standardized method of measurement, evaluation, and feedback.

6. Publisher: Consulting Psychologist Press, Inc.
577 College Avenue
Palo Alto, CA 94306

D. Basic Skills Screening Test

1. Purpose: A test designed to objectively test target behaviors and suggest remediation activities for mentally retarded and handicapped individuals.

2. Description: Assesses 7 categories of skills: sensory-motor functioning, visual processing, auditory processing, language, symbolic operation, social-emotional development, and work skills.

3. Administration: Administered individually through direct interaction with the client. Can be administered by teachers.

4. Technical Data: Standardized.

5. Additional Comments: A screening test that identifies deficit skill areas and provides teaching objectives, remediation activities, materials, and profile sheet.

6. Publisher: Mid-Nebraska Mental Retardation Services
518 Eastside Boulevard
Hastings, NE 68901

E. Behavioral Characteristics Progression (1973)

1. Purpose: The BCP is a criterion-referenced observational tool that is intended for assessment of mentally and behaviorally exceptional children.

2. Description: This instrument is a nonstandardized continuum of behaviors in chart form. It involves assessment of existing behaviors and can be used to derive appropriate objectives. The BCP consists of 2400 observable traits referred to as behavioral characteristics grouped into categories of behaviors called behavior strands.

3. Administration: Can be administered by a teacher, team, or child care workers. Administered by direct observation.

4. Technical Data: Not standardized.

5. Additional Comments: The BCP serves as a communication tool among staff members because a child's status is easily observed by all. It contains strands particularly appropriate for the deaf, blind, and orthopedically handicapped.

6. Publisher: VORT Corporation
P. O. Box 11132
Palo Alto, CA 94306

F. Behavioral Developmental Profile

   1. Purpose: This profile was devised to assist in the assessment of handicapped and culturally deprived children between the ages of birth to 6 years.

   2. Description: The test consists of developmental skills in the following 3 areas: communication, motor, and social. This profile also provides a total age score.

   3. Administration: Familiarity with the test material is all that is needed to administer this test. Test materials consist of a manual and a protocol sheet. No other materials are needed for the assessment.

   4. Technical Data: Not standardized.

   5. Additional Comments: This instrument provides information on behavioral objectives and strategies which would assist in the development of programming for the child. This profile is not restricted to any particular population.

   6. Publisher: Marshalltown Project
Attn: J. Montgomery
507 East Anson
Marshalltown, OH 50158

G. Denver Developmental Screening Test

   1. Purpose: This test was designed to detect delays and abnormalities in normal development for children between birth and 6 years of age.

   2. Description: The DDST is comprised of 105 items written in range of accomplishments. These items are arranged on the test in the following four sections: personal-social, fine motor, adaptive,

language, gross motor. A bar on the test profile indicates the ages at which 25%, 50%, 75%, and 90% of normal children are able to perform particular items.

3. Administration: This test can be administered by persons with no special training in psychological testing. The child is tested on 20 sample items; some parental reporting is accepted.

4. Technical Data: The DDST was standardized on 1000 normal children in the Denver area to see at what ages they could do each of the items.

5. Additional Comments: This is a simple, useful tool to aid in the discovery of children with developmental problems.

6. Publisher: The LaDoca Company, Project and Publishing Foundation, Inc.
East 51st and Lincoln
Denver, CO 80216

H. The Developmental Record
    1. Purpose: This instrument is designed as a convenient instrument which can be used by various levels of observers to obtain a rapid descriptive picture of individual functioning and progress along a developmental continuum.

    2. Description: The DR is intended for use with developmentally delayed individuals and contains 5 major developmental sections: self-care, perceptual-motor, social, communication, and self-direction. Seven additional scales are provided under optional designa-

	tion for handicapped or behavioral problems.
3. Administration:	Can be administered by a teacher, trained aides, or parents. Items are marked if it is known that the individual can perform them; if it is not known how the individual will perform, he or she is tested on particular items in question.
4. Technical Data:	Standardized.
5. Additional Comments:	The primary focus is on the identification of developmental benchmarks. Three levels of independence are suggested: (a) dependence (roughly normal development up to 1 1/2 years); (b) semi-independent (roughly 2 to 5 1/2 years); and (c) independent (roughly 6 years to maturity).
6. Publisher:	Continuing Education Publications 1633 Southwest Park Avenue Box 1491 Portland, OR 97207

I. Developmental Scales: To be used in assessing the development of deaf-blind children

1. Purpose:	This is a developmental scale to be used for the assessment of deaf-blind and multi-handicapped children.
2. Description:	This instrument is comprised of 177 items in the following major areas of development: personal, self-help, social, gross motor, fine motor, communication, visual, and cognitive development.

3. Administration: To be administered by the classroom teacher through direct observation.

4. Technical Data: Not standardized.

5. Additional Comments: This scale was compiled from several existing scales and from observation of deaf-blind children. The format was designed to serve as a means of obtaining baseline data appropriate for use by teachers in the classroom setting. The 7 major areas covered represent samples of the various critical behaviors in the child's development.

6. Publisher: Mountain Plains Regional Center for Handicapped Children
165 Cook Street
Denver, CO 80206

J. Education for Multi-handicapped Infants Assessment Scale

1. Purpose: This scale is intended to provide information to direct individualized planning for infants; results can be translated into instructional objectives.

2. Description: This scale is intended for use with multi-handicapped infants, birth to 2 years. It provides for evaluation of functioning in the following areas of development: gross motor, fine motor, socialization, cognition, and language.

3. Administration: To be administered by a teacher through direct observation.

4. Technical Data: Not standardized.

5. Additional Comments: This instrument can be used as a checklist for the individualized, diagnostic, and prescriptive

<table>
<tr><td></td><td>teaching of infants. Is easily administered, concise, and has a color-coded scale.</td></tr>
<tr><td>6. Publisher:</td><td>Department of Pediatrics
University of Virginia Medical Center
Box 232
Charlottesville, VA 22901</td></tr>
</table>

K. Fairview Behavior Evaluation Battery

1. Purpose:	The Fairview Battery is designed for use with the mildly, moderately, severely, and profoundly retarded individuals. This scale is particularly applicable to low functioning persons.
2. Description:	This battery consists of 5 scales designed to measure behaviors and skills among all levels of retarded individuals from birth to 10 years and older. Each of the following scales is short and easily administered: developmental scale, self-help scale, social skills scale, language evaluation scale, problem behavior record.
3. Administration:	Any persons, such as a teacher, parent, or caretaker, can administer this scale. The observer circles the number preceding the statement which best describes the individual's typical behavior.
4. Technical Data:	This scale was standardized on the mentally retarded at the Fairview State Hospital in California.
5. Additional Comments:	The developmental scale may be used to measure improvement in

individuals or groups.

6. Publisher: Fairview State Hospital
Research Department
2501 Harbor Boulevard
Costa Mesa, CA 92626

L. Koontz Child Developmental Program

     1. Purpose: An evaluation program for normal children who are developmentally between 0 to 48 months.

     2. Description: The Koontz provides for evaluation of performance in the areas of gross motor, fine motor, social, and language.

     3. Administration: Administered individually by direct observation of and/or performance of items after one week of observation. Begin where child is, rather than at the beginning of each section.

     4. Technical Data: Standardized.

     5. Additional Comments: In addition to the evaluation, the Koontz provides training activities to help train skills for each month from 1 to 48.

     6. Publisher: Western Psychological Services Publishers and Distributors
12031 Wilshire Boulevard
Los Angeles, CA 90025

M. Lakeland Village Adaptive Behavior Grid

     1. Purpose: This is a criterion-referenced test that is to serve as a diagnostic tool to assist in the assessment of mentally handicapped children; the developmental scales range from birth to 10 years of age.

     2. Description: The grid provides a graphic description of the child's strengths and weaknesses in the following

categories: eating, toileting, dressing, health, communication, ability, vocational aptitude, socialization, orientation, and behavior control.

3. Administration: This test is not timed, and familiarity with the test materials is all that is needed in administering the assessment device.

4. Technical Data: Not standardized.

5. Additional Comments: This is a developmental scale; the items provide an age-value score. Thus, the child can be compared with standards of adaptive behavior found in the community. It can also assist in the establishment of programming goals.

6. Publisher: Lakeland Village
Medical Lake, WA 99022

N. Learning Accomplishment Profile for the Young Child

1. Purpose: The LAP is designed to provide the teacher of the young handicapped child with a criterion-referenced record of his existing skills. Appropriate for multi-handicapped populations.

2. Description: The manual contains 3 sections:
Behavioral — provides a basis of evaluation of the child's existing skills in 6 areas: gross motor, fine motor, social, self-help, cognitive, and language.
Task Analysis — provides guidance in sequencing skill development and a system of recording responses on a specific task.
Unit Development — contains

	44 weeks of curriculum units in ready-made teaching sequence.
3. Administration:	Can be administered by teachers. Child is tested on items and by direct observation.
4. Technical Data:	Not standardized.
5. Additional Comments:	The LAP enables the teacher to identify developmentally appropriate learning objectives for each child, measure progress through changes in the rate of development, and provide specific information relevant to pupil learning.
6. Publisher:	Chapel Hill Training-Outreach Project Lincoln Center, Merritt Mill Chapel Hill, NC 27514

O. A Manual for the Assessment of a Deaf-Blind, Multiply Handicapped Child, Revised edition.

1. Purpose:	This scale was developed to approximate the early developmental sequence of deaf-blind children. It is suggested that this instrument be administered twice yearly over a 3-year period to measure growth.
2. Description:	The components of this scale contain the following areas: personal self-help, social development, gross motor development, fine motor development, language, and cognition. Each area contains items which are marked when the child can do them. Space is provided for initial evaluation and 5 subsequent assessments.
3. Administration:	Can be administered by a class-

room teacher through direct observation.

4. Technical Data: Not standardized.

5. Additional Comments: This scale is reported to reflect the development of deaf-blind children more accurately than do scales for children without sensory impairments.

6. Publisher: Midwest Regional Center for Services to Deaf-Blind Children
P. O. Box 420
Lansing, MI 48902

P. Pennsylvania Training Model, Individual Assessment Guide

1. Purpose: A competency checklist designed for use with multi-handicapped public school children.

2. Description: A planning system designed for use by teachers to assist in the development of specific programs for the multi-handicapped. Consists of a gross assessment in major areas and a specific assessment within areas.

3. Administration: Administered by the classroom teacher through direct observation.

4. Technical Data: Not standardized.

5. Additional Comments: Its use provides a broad assessment of the individual's total needs. Can be used for the severely and profoundly retarded as well as the multi-handicapped.

6. Publisher: Dr. Duffy, Regional Resource Center
443 S. Gulph Road
King of Prussia, PA 19406

Q. A Programmatic Guide to Assessing Severely/Profoundly

Handicapped Children

1. Purpose:	This scale provides a checklist of normative developmental sequencing about the child being assessed. The assessment device has scales ranging from birth to 5 years of age.
2. Description:	The Progammatic Guide provides information pertaining to the child's functional level in each of the following areas: self-help skills, communication skills, gross motor skills, fine motor skills, sensory discrimination, preacademics, and prereading skills.
3. Administration:	This test requires only that someone familiar with the child observe his various behavioral patterns. It requires that a rater check observable behavioral responses.
4. Technical Data:	Not standardized.
5. Additional Comments:	This device was created to assist educators in assessing severely and profoundly handicapped children. Can help in establishing educational goals for individual children. The increments of the scale are very detailed and sensitive to behavioral changes; they also provide information as to next higher criteria to be taught.
6. Publisher:	Experimental Educational Unit Child Development and Mental Retardation Center University of Washington Seattle, WA 98195

R. Project MEMPHIS Instruments for Individual Program Planning and Evaluation (Comprehensive Developmental Scale)

1. Purpose: A developmental scale designed for use with children with a developmental age between 3 months and 5 years of age.

2. Description: A developmental evaluation can be provided in the areas of: personal-social skills, gross motor skills, fine motor skills, language skills, and perceptual-cognitive skills.

3. Administration: This is an easily administered scale that can be given by the classroom teacher. The method of assessment is direct observation.

4. Technical Data: Not standardized.

5. Additional Comments: The MEMPHIS yields a developmental age for a child in each of the five above-mentioned areas.

6. Publisher: Fearon Publishers
6 Davis Drive
Belmont, CA 94002

S. RADEA: Teaching Manual; Testing and Remediation

1. Purpose: This instrument is intended for training behaviors of students who are functioning between the developmental ages of 0 to 7 years.

2. Description: The RADEA materials represent a program placement test for students entering a special education program. The following components are assessed: visual perception, auditory perception, perceptual motor, oral langauge, functional living.

3. Administration: Can be administered by the classroom teacher through direct observation.

4. Technical Data: Not standardized.

5. Additional Comments: A unique feature of this system is the availability of a rental inservice program to train persons in the use of RADEA materials.

6. Publisher: Melton Book Company, Inc.
                        111 Leslie
                        Dallas, TX 75207

T. TMR Performance Profile for the Severely and Moderately Retarded

1. Purpose: A scale designed for rating the skills for severely multi-handicapped children who have developed some level of independence.

2. Description: This scale includes ratings in the areas of: social behavior, self-care, communication, basic knowledge, practical skills, and body usage.

3. Administration: An easy to administer scale that can be given by a teacher or paraprofessional. Method of assessment is through observation of the child in various behavioral situations.

4. Technical Data: A criterion-referenced test.

5. Additional Comments: There is a profile sheet for summary of scores in each area. Each item in major areas is rated from 0 to 4 depending upon level of competence.

6. Publisher: Educational Performance Associates
                        563 Westview Avenue
                        Ridgefield, NJ 07657

U. Vineland Social Maturity Scale

1. Purpose:	This scale is designed to measure the level of social maturity of individuals from birth to maturity. It can provide information pertaining to any type of handicapped individual.
2. Description:	A checklist of skills attained at yearly intervals in the areas of self-help, communication, self-direction, socialization, locomotion, and occupation.
3. Administration:	The test requires only that the examiner interview someone who is familiar with the individual being assessed or that the examiner be familiar with the subject. Qualifications to administer the test are minimal, but it is mandatory that the examiner understand the criteria as established by the manual.
4. Technical Data:	The Vineland Scale is a standardized scale which provides normative data. Various maturational and behavioral criteria are established.
5. Additional Comments:	The test provides an age equivalent score and a social quotient. These two scores are said to relate to mental age and intelligence quotient.
6. Publisher:	American Guidance Service, Inc. Publishers Building Circle Pines, MN 55014

CHAPTER EIGHT

VOCATIONAL EVALUATION ISSUES/ PROCEDURES WITH THE SEVERE AND MULTI-HANDICAPPED POPULATION

MIKE ROSS, ED.D.

PREVOCATIONAL CONSIDERATIONS FOR THE SEVERELY AND MULTI-HANDICAPPED

MOST of the facilities serving this population have historically defined their goals in terms of preparing their clients for vocational placement. Thus, an assumption is made that readiness is a critical factor in various prevocational skill areas such as social functioning, fine and gross motor skills, and self-help skills. Generally, skills in these various areas are then task analyzed and identified as prerequisites for entering sheltered workshops. Consequently, these skills, such as sorting or folding, retraining in self-help, community living, or language skills, are taught under the assumption that they are necessary for later vocational success. The practice of labeling these skills are prerequisites for vocational training implies that individuals who are incapable of performing these skills will not be able to master later vocational tasks. However, a large body of contemporary research that has assessed the vocational potential of the severely and multi-handicapped has contradicted this notion that many such prevocational skills are necessary precursers to later vocational success (Bellamy et al., 1975; Gold, 1973; 1975; 1976; Gold, 1).

The fact that individuals with minimal self-help skills, minimal language, and no previous systematic vocational training have been able to learn complex skills and exhibit competence in these skills over an extended period of time suggests a different role for both prevocational training and vocational assessment. The obvious implication from this for prevocational training would be for those individuals involved with the pre-vocational training of this population to simply identify those skills that are most crucial in the workshop environment and then systematically teach them. The clear implication from these findings for the practice of vocational assessment for the severely and multi-handicapped is to again identify the most crucial or most commonly used skills in various jobs, assess those skills, and not worry about tangential or inconsequential skills not important for various kinds of jobs.

Horner and Bellamy (1978) indicate that the best way to improve the utilities of teaching prevocational skills is to teach skills that extend beyond the specific examples or settings used in the instruction rather than teaching specific responses to specific stimuli. This is a teaching methodology that Becker and Engleman (1977) refer to as teaching a "general case." Becker and Engleman define a general case as having been taught when, after instruction on some tasks in a particular class, any task in that class can be performed correctly. In the context of prevocational training, then, Horner and Bellamy would view the teaching of the general case as identifying the most commonly used concepts and operations that a worker encounters and teachs as generalized skills. Horner and Bellamy see this as a two-step process: first the task that would be needed in a specific workshop or school program situation should be identified; and second, the concepts and operations most used across those tasks should be identified. For example, the most commonly used skills in areas such as tool use (e.g. pliers, screwdriver) for basic assembly (e.g. screwing a bolt, using a bend setup to sequence assembly parts) would have to be identified and taught in a variety of contexts so that maximum generalization would be obtained. This is a very important consideration because a certain amount of training will always be necessary in a workshop situation even if the individual can perform most of the component parts of certain skills.

Finally, the distinction between vocational and prevocational training is not as distinct as many professionals in the field seem to believe. As Gold and Pomerantz (1978) indicate, the differences between vocational and prevocational training and programming are for the most part arbitrary. Since no areas of instruction are purely vocational, prevocational, or nonvocational, the important issue is one of general good programming and curriculum in each of these areas.

VOCATIONAL ASSESSMENT FOR THE SEVERELY AND MULTI-HANDICAPPED

The dynamics involved in a vocational assessment are the same as those related to "general" assessment and assessment for academic and curriculum purposes. Thus, the discussion of the various dynamics involved in the process of assessment is in order.

Criterion Referenced Approaches

The criterion reference approach to testing is one of evaluating an individual's performance to an absolute criterion for that particular subject instead of comparing his performance to that of a standardized or normative group. Recognition of the individual's performance is not based on what others have done at a certain age scale or point scale, but on the number of items performed by the subject. The subject is either able to perform at mastery or instructional level or is simply not ready for that given task. Through the process of elimination, the examiner can identify where that individual should be functioning. Mastery level may consist of the subject being able to do 90 percent of the material or objectives given to him on a given task, while instructional level is at 70 percent, and any performance below that point is considered frustration level performance. It must be emphasized here that the decision of 85, 90, or 95 percent for Mastery or 65 or 70 percent for instructional level is a purely arbitrary decision on the part of the examiner.

The biggest difficulty with this type of testing is the examiner's ability to assess from the client's records in past experiences what set of criteria should be used and what the appropriate methods of presentation to the subject should be. Another problem is in the recognition of the client's ability to handle certain situations and yet not be able to cope or work in another type of setting.

Norm Referenced Approaches

Norm reference testing of the severely and multi-handicapped client for vocational roles is one of defining task analysis assessment. In essence, what is task analyzed or defined is how one handicapped individual with certain characteristics compares with another individual with similar characteristics.

Norm reference devices are those tests that compare the subject's performance to the performance of his group. The prevocational assessment of a multi-handicapped child would be one of learning which child has what skill and where that particular child fits into a rank order of how to perform on different scale items. The skill items or tasks would be set to either a point scale or an age scale ranking. Salvia and Ysseldyke (1978) relate that age scales are developed by scaling test items in terms of the percentages of children of different ages responding correctly to each test item. They also relate that a point scale is constructed by selecting and ordering items of different levels of difficulty.

Norm referenced assessments are such that their results indicate a person's performance in a standardized set for groups of individuals and should be administered by a well-trained specialist. The norm referenced device allows the examiner to compare the examinee's performance to that of many others without testing all the others in any given time span.

The norm referenced assessment, however, does not allow for or supply a built-in adjusted score for developmental differences from one subject to the next. It more or less relies on the competence of the examiner to adjust or recognize these differences. Little consideration is made for the examinee in reference from one skill to the next if he has not passed a specified number of skills within the sequence.

Although norm referenced tests allow for a standardized placement and usually take less time, because some tests can be given in group fashion and others have set time variables, they do have their limitations and are only as good as the examiner who is administering them. They are objective and have predetermined answers and standards for the examiner's use. However, if the examiner is not in full control and does not have the ability to recognize the test's shortcomings and the examinee's limitations, poor interpretation of the results may follow.

One-shot vs. On-going Evaluation

As Brolin (1976) indicates, psychologists have tended to view diagnosing the mentally retarded as a test-and-run situation. This test-and-run syndrome is particularly disastrous when one considers Neff's (1970) comment that the measurement of human behavior is not as straightforward as the measurement of physical objects or energies. He further indicates that psychological assessment presents three problems: (1) it is impossible to fix the unit of measurement, therefore, it is more of an ordering process (e.g. a person with an IQ of 100 does not necessarily have twice the ability of an individual with an IQ of 50); (2) the inherent unpredictability of psychological behaviors; and (3) it is very indirect and occurs before the fact. These same inherent problems of psychological assessment certainly exist in the area of vocational evaluation also.

One-shot evaluations leave much to be desired because they only allow the subject to be seen in one set of circumstances at one particular point in time. The examiner himself is not totally capable of ascertaining whether he has chosen the correct test materials or even the proper setting to make judgments on that given subject. Too many variables are left to chance on a one-shot assessment. The examiner cannot adjust for all possible variables as he could with an on-going evaluation.

The variables could affect the scores, or they may not be important at all. However, the evaluator must be aware of the variables and be able to take them into consideration. The examiner must be aware of "who the subject is:" his physical limitations, conditions of his immediate dominating environment, his attitude, his feelings of testing and of the examiner, his physical and mental health at the time of the assessment, his response rate, and his level of understanding. The physical limitations of the assessment must be appropriate for a reliable score and performance.

The on-going evaluation allows the evaluator time for a thorough investigation and retesting of specific skill areas with different assessment techniques, which a one-shot evaluation would not allow. The evaluator is able to compensate for irregularities within a testing situation (e.g. emotional trauma or unexpected interruption) and can make adjustments for the physical environment if it is inappropriate at any given time.

The on-going evaluation also allows the existing attitude and moods of the evaluator to change. Examiners are human too and react differently under different sets of stimuli in environmental pressures. An evaluator's patience and understanding are at various levels at various times. Even though the tasks may be "objective," too often the evaluator's subjective moods could alter the results.

The on-going evaluation permits the evaluator to make behavioral observations over a longer period of time and reaffirms the scores of prior testing to match consistent behavior. These scores would then be more of a predictive agent rather than a one-shot estimate of what the client's performance on a particular task will be, based on results of a certain test battery.

The on-going evaluation also allows the client's instructor to be aware of and better monitor his progress and to be able to restate and adjust other short- and long-term goals of a client's specific behavioral/educational/vocational plan.

Informal vs. Formal Assessment Techniques

The informal assessment can be a highly useful tool in the evaluation of daily activities of the severely and multi-handicapped individuals. The evaluator or instructor on an informal basis can determine quickly and effectively where the individual is at a point in time, based on prior test measures and the individual's present performance. The evaluator or instructor has to be aware of the limits of his ability to diagnose the performance of the client in terms of his training or instrumentation limitations.

If the instructor is skilled, he will be able to diagnose and evaluate his own effectiveness by the performance of the individual. The individual will be able to gain more insight and knowledge because the instructor will be able to plan and operate the habilitative program in tune with the client's development.

The formal testing should be completed by the examiner who has been trained in the administration of that particular assessment tool. The formal testing allows the instructor of the individual to have a starting/reference point to work from at the beginning of the client's habilitative program. The formal testing can provide an in-depth picture of the handicapped individual's total functioning ability. Informal assessment only allows for a one-shot behavioral/academic skill assessment, which will be used in developing a short-term goal, while the formal assessment provides the examiner with an overall picture and provides the instructor with material that will provide information to project long-term goals. With the assistance of the evaluator, the instructor can then interpret the results of formal assessment evaluation and adapt them to his planning program for each individual. This plan then provides educational/performance checkpoints which the instructor can use in an informal assessment to check the client's gains.

Thus, one can see that both the formal and informal use of testing have proper places and, if used wisely, can provide for highly productive programs for the client and instructor.

ESTABLISHING ASSESSMENT PRIORITIES

In Relation to Future Role of Client

In considering future role of the client in the work force, one must keep in mind the point emphasized by Pomerantz and Marholen (1977) that even if normative vocational assessment data is valid and reliable, it is not particularly useful for the individual who will have no opportunity to join the labor force in the "mainstream" of society. Pomerantz and Marholen further remind us that even though evaluators may be among the most highly trained and skilled individuals in a workshop setting, they spend considerable time and energy collecting data that has a high probability of not being used. They further suggest that it may be far more productive to have these staff members engaged in potentially more productive activities, such as job placement and specific skill training. Another important factor to keep in mind, in establishing assessment priorities in using the results of assessment, is that the practice of vocational evaluation of severely and multi-handicapped individuals in and of itself certainly does not lead to the solution of their problems (Gold 1975). It is certainly a questionable practice to obtain a lot of data in relation to the potential of severely and multi-handicapped clients to perform more complex kinds of tasks if these kinds of tasks are not required or included in their specific workshop situation. In addition to this practice, attention given to the modification and/or training of new and more complex social adjustment skills is of little value if the client is never put in a work environment that requires these more complex skills; perhaps the time would be much better spent in teaching specific skills that would be needed in a particular workshop situation.

In Relation to Cost, Time, and Personnel Consideration

Paulson (1978), in a discussion of the Views Evaluation System, indicated that it, like any other system, is only as good as the people using it. He emphasized the importance of follow-up after evaluation, suggesting that if adequate follow-up is not undertaken the evaluation report will take its place in the student's file along with a lot of other useless documents. However, if used appropriately, the vocational evaluation with adequate follow-up affords the instructors, parents, and employers valuable information that can enhance the client's vocational success. The practice of having a professional do nothing but evaluations is a gross misuse of this human resource. The practice of specific skill evaluation certainly has its place, but its value is badly diluted if it is not supplemented by an effort on the part of the evaluator to do adequate work on follow-up with instructors, employers, and parents. Perhaps the best rule of thumb to use in making sure the cost, time, and personnel considerations are used wisely is to simply not evaluate a client in specific skill areas where it is not likely that the client will have the opportunity to use these skills.

SPECIFIC VOCATIONAL EVALUATION METHODS

Although there are many methods and techniques of vocational evaluation, they all have the same goals in mind — the matching of appropriate vocational goals in relation to a client's specific occupational and work abilities and behavior. The writers, then, view vocational evaluation in the context of the United States Department of Health, Education and Welfare (1971) definition: "the appraisal of the individual's capacity including patterns of work behavior ability to acquire occupational skills, and the selection of appropriate vocational goals" (p. 1). The major techniques of vocational evaluation are standardized tests, behavior checklists or rating scales, work samples, and situational assessment.

Standardized Psychological Tests

Standardized psychological tests generally are designed to measure skills in a restricted context; for example, dexterity, perception, achievement, interests, personality, and aptitude. Although standardized psychological tests of various types are very widely used for industrial selection and appraisal in industries and workshops, they have met with very little success with the severely and multi-handicapped because these individuals usually score below the norms established for these tests. Indeed, most standardized psychological tests have fallen well short of expectations even with the normal population. Standardized psychological tests used in industry and workshops may, in some instances, have respectably high reliability, but very low predictive validity (Neff, 1968; Burrows Mental Measurements Yearbook, 1978). These tests have been found to have particularly limited value with mentally retarded individuals with little or no work history, thus requiring the extensive use of alternative methods of work assessment (Neff, 1968; Flexer and Martin, 1978).

Despite these serious limitations, standardized psychological tests of one form or another are still used extensively by various schools and agencies concerned with vocational training of the severely and multi-handicapped. As Overs (1970) indicates, the continued use of various standardized tests, particularly of manual dexterity, exists because many believe that these tests predict future success in specific vocational tasks as well as or better than job sample tasks and are considerably more efficient in terms of simplicity of administration and saving of client and staff time.

Bennet Hand Tool Dexterity Test

The Bennet Hand Tool Dexterity Test (Psychological Corporation, New York) is a measure of competency in using common mechanics tools. This test, which consists of a wooden frame with two uprights extending from a horizontal base, measures mechanical aptitude in the use of common tools. There are three rows containing three holes on each upright in which the client must insert nine bolts, washers, and nut units using such tools as an adjustable wrench and a screwdriver. The client must then transfer the bolts, nuts, and washers to the other side as quickly as possible while fastening them together. The directions on this test are rather detailed; thus, this population may have some trouble understanding and following the directions. However, the format does permit the supplementation of directions by the examiner.

Crawford Small Parts Dexterity Test

This test, designed to measure eye-hand coordination, consists of a board containing forty-two holes on the left and right bottom and three bins for pins, collars, and screws on the top. Tweezers must be used to pick up one pin, place this pin in a hole in the board, and fit the collar over the pin. The individual must then use a screw driver to put thirty screws in a plate after the completion of the thirty-six pins and collars. This test requires no reading, and the client's scores are recorded by the amount of time required to complete the task.

Purdue Pegboard

The Purdue Pegboard (Science Research Associates) is a widely used test designed to assess manual dexterity for industrial jobs. The pegboard contains two rows, each with twenty-five holes into which pins are inserted. There are four cups containing pins, washers, and collars at the top of the board. An assessment is made of bi-manual dexterity and right- and left-hand dexterity separately. Both manual dexterity and finger dexterity are assessed in this test. Reading ability is not required for this test and it is simple to administer and score.

Minnesota Weight of Manipulation Test

The Minnesota Weight of Manipulation Test (Western Psychological Services) contains five subtests, each assessing a different manipulative ability, e.g. placing, turning, displacing, and single and bi-manual turning. The format is a form board containing sixty round holes and sixty discs that must be placed into the holes. Although somewhat time-consuming, this test is rather easy to administer and score. In addition, many retarded individuals seem to enjoy taking this test.

Pennsylvania Bi-manual Work Sample

This test, as the name implies, is an assessment of bi-manual manipulative ability. The format consists of a two and one-half foot long board, which contains fifty holes on one side, and a bin on the opposite side, which contains fifty nuts and bolts. In the middle of this form board are five rows containing ten holes each into which the assembled nut and bolt is placed in an upside-down position. The client is required to assemble and then disassemble the nuts and bolts. Both workshop and industrial norms exist for this test. The test is flexible in terms of accommodating an individual who is right-handed or left-handed. It is very simple to administer and is enjoyed by the retarded clients who take it.

Non-reading Interest Test

The use of non-reading pictorial interest tests has gained wide use with the mentally retarded and multi-handicapped population in recent years. Obviously, assessing vocational interests with the moderate severely retarded and multi-handicapped population is a very difficult task. However, if used wisely, various non-reading vocational interests tests can have considerable utility when used with the moderately retarded population. The following are representative of some non-reading vocational interest surveys that could be used with this population.

Geist Picture Interest Inventory

The Geist Picture Interest Inventory (Western Psychological Corporation), which assesses interest in eleven areas, is used widely in sheltered workshop and other rehabilitation assessment. Each of the forty-four items on the test consist of three drawings depicting specific job activities with captions under each depicting various client preferences (e.g. "Which would you rather do for a living?").

Program for Assessing Youth Employment Skills (Payes)

The Payes (Educational Testing Service, Princeton, New Jersey) is a comprehensive, three-part inventory which assesses a number of vocationally-relevant factors in the following areas: how people should act on a job (11 items), attitude toward supervisors (13 items), self-confidence (15 items), and interest inventory (28 items), job knowledge (30 items), job seeking skills (17 items), and practical reasoning (20 items). Due to the complexity of the items involved on the Payes, it would only have utility with individuals functioning in the moderate to mild range of retardation who have possibilities for outside employment.

Vocational Interests and Sophistication Assessment (VISA)

This reading-free inventory purports to assess the vocational interests of the mentally retarded in terms of specific areas of interest and knowledge of job conditions. Separate versions of the VISA exist for males and females. For the males, the inventory consists of a series of seventy-five pictures that depict seven job clusters (food service, garage, laundry, farm and grounds, light industrial, maintenance and material handling). The female version contains fifty-three items or pictures that deal with four job clusters (food service, business clerical, housekeeping, and laundry) (Parnicky, Kahn, and Burdett, 1964).

Areas included in the inventory are sophistication inquiry, responses to questions to each of the job areas; explaining the task (identifying figures used in the various items) and interest inquiries (the client expressing preferences for jobs depicted in various pictures). The authors have obtained adequate standardization data.

Reading-Free Vocational Interests Inventory

This inventory is based on job profiles contained in the *Guide to Jobs for the Mentally Retarded* (Peterson and Jones, 1964). This inventory, like the VISA, contains separate versions for males and females. The male version contains eleven job clusters scales (building trade, automotive, animal care, clerical, food service, patient care, horticulture, janitorial, personal service, laundry service, and materials handling). The female version contains eight cluster scales (laundry, clerical, light industrial, personal service, food service, horticulture, patient care, and housekeeping). Each scale contains fifteen items and the client is required to indicate preference from three pictures. The client's preference for each interest area is indicated in the percentile fashion in relation to the number of times he selects items that are key to a specific area. This inventory could have some utility with individuals functioning in the moderate to mild range of retardation. Like other interest inventories, significant modifications in terms of speed and manner of presentation may have to be made by the examiner.

Vocational Behavior Checklists

Various types of checklists or rating scales are used extensively in industrial, sheltered workshop, and rehabilitation settings. The use of various types of formal behavior checklists have gained widespread use in rehabilitative settings in recent years because professionals have assumed that these instruments offer a more valid and objective means of evaluating client skills. However, this is not necessarily true, particularly if the professional does not take into account some crucial factors that would indicate how appropriate a particular instrument would be for a specific client.

The rehabilitation professional should have established criteria in mind before selecting a particular vocational behavior checklist. The need for using a particular behavior checklist could vary considerably in relation to different needs of the checklist user, e.g. such factors as the ability level of a client, placement options and facilities available, and time and training of the examiner. Walls and Werner (1977) describe and rate a series of vocational behavior checklists according to what they feel are four crucial criteria: scope, objectivity, setting, and prescriptive-descriptive factors. Scope is seen as the total number of vocational items and number of different subclasses represented. The criteria for objectivity is how observable or behavioral the checklist items are. Setting merely refers to the environment or situation in which the client is expected to demonstrate specific skills, e.g. a training class, on the job, or both. A checklist with descriptive items is defined in which the client's current skill repertoire is the major consideration. A checklist containing prescriptive items describes procedures for training a skill.

Walls and Werner found that the behavior checklist that they reviewed varied considerably in relation to these four criteria. Some checklists would rate very high on one or two of these criterias, such as scope and objectivity, and be weak in the other areas. Because no one behavior checklist meets high standards in each of these four areas, Wall and Werner suggest that one useful strategy might be to select various items from subclasses of different behavior checklists. In this way, one could selectively compile items to increase both objectivity and scope.

One critical point for the rehabilitation professional to keep in mind in the use of checklists is to remember that the primary reason for their use is to systematically assess individual competencies. The efficacious use of vocational behavior checklists can serve as a valuable tool for curriculum planning and revision of programs. However, vocational behavior checklists are not training programs in themselves. In addition, they should be used in conjunction with many other types of vocational assessment before making critical decisions affecting the client's future and welfare.

A comprehensive description of a large number of behavior checklists is contained in an annotated bibliography by Wall, Werner, Bacon, and Zane (1977). Following is a brief discussion of some selected behavior rating scales.

AAMD Adaptive Behavior Scale

The public school version of the AAMD Adaptive Behavior Scale was designed for the use of school personnel in order to evaluate the individual's adaptive behavior and make recommendations for specific areas where remediation is needed. The scale is to provide a realistic point of reference for the child's behavior within his environment and his response to that environment.

The AAMD Adaptive Behavior Scale is divided into two major sections. The first section is an evaluation along developmental lines. The child's behavior is evaluated in ten major areas: (a) independent functioning, (b) physical development, (c) economic activity, (d) language development, (e) numbers and time, (f) domestic activity, (g) vocational activity, (h) self-direction, (i) responsibility, and (j) socialization.

The second section of the AAMD public school version supplies the examiner with the information in regard to the individual's maladaptive behavior related to personality and behavior disorders. This section of the AAMD consists of fourteen parts: (a) violent and destructive behavior, (b) anti-social behavior, (c) rebellious behavior, (d) untrustworthy behavior, (e) withdrawal, (f) stereotype behavior and odd mannerisms, (g) inappropriate interpersonal manners, (h) unacceptable vocal habits, (i) unacceptable or eccentric habits, (j) self-abusive behavior, (k) hyperactive tendencies, (1) sexually aberrant behavior, (m) psychological disturbances, and (n) use of medications.

The time element with the AAMD when using the interview method takes fifteen to twenty minutes. The scale is administered on an individual basis. The third party interview using the parent is the advisable method for completion of this scale.

Social and Prevocational Information Battery (SPIB)

The SPIB was developed to assess the mildly retarded individual's ability to function within the community in the following areas: (a) employability, (b) economic self-sufficiency, (c) family living, (d) personal habits, and (e) communication. The five areas are tested via nine subtests and each subtest has its own content area. These content areas are the following: (a) job search skills, (b) job related behavior, (c) banking, (d) budgeting, (e) purchasing habits, (f) home management, (g) physical health care, (h) hygiene and grooming, and (i) functional signs.

The test is given in an oral format and the student responds to true and false questions. The testing can be divided into nine segments, with one segment for each subtest. Testing in each area should be in twenty to thirty minute periods. The number of individuals being tested should not exceed ten. This test minimizes reading skill ability on the part of the client — enabling him to express himself through his answers without being penalized because of poor reading ability.

The writers feel that this test could be modified to meet the needs of the moderately retarded adult. The major modification would consist primarily of giving very careful attention to the language and time variables, i.e. simplifying the terms used in administering the battery and spreading out the subtests. Items that are too difficult or thought to be inappropriate for this population would simply be eliminated in the administration of the SPIB to these populations. Of course, one would have to keep these actions in mind in considering the client's performance on this battery.

Situational Assessment

A structured situational assessment strategy is used to critically evaluate the client's capacity to adjust to various social demands of work tasks and work environments. Such factors as the client's motivation, preferences, reactions to distracting stimuli, and perseverance can be assessed via situational assessment. The most common type of situational assessment is a job try-out. In the job try-out format the client is placed in a controlled work setting that is closely monitored in order to determine the nature of his responses to this setting, various types and degrees of supervision, types of work tasks, and response to peers (Gellman, 1970).

A structured situational assessment strategy can yield many benefits in evaluating the work functioning and/or potential of a severely and multi-handicapped. A good behavioral observation can provide baseline data that could serve as a foundation for an individual program plan. In addition, a structured behavioral assessment technique can be helpful in determining curriculum priorities. However, as Gold (1978) indicates, a behavioral assessment can only be truly useful to the evaluator or instructor if it focuses on the specific behaviors prerequisite to a target task. Evaluating only general behavioral constructs is not viewed by Gold as useful because it does not focus the instructor's attention on specific skills and hence does not yield data useful to further instruction.

The writers feel that a structured situation observation should meet two requirements: (1) it should enable the evaluator/trainer to pinpoint a precise description of behavior, and (2) it should allow for accurate specification of the rate of a particular behavior.

The following is a simple, quick and inexpensive method of situational assessment that can be used in most settings; vocational classroom, sheltered workshop or job placement site. This procedure can be used with a single individual or with a group of up to twelve evaluees. The only special equipment required is a stop watch (a timer, clock or watch) and some simple forms.

ESTABLISH TASK NORMS. The first step is to conduct a

standard time study on the task to be performed. Preferably the time study should be conducted with not less than three non-handicapped individuals. These individuals should become thoroughly familiar with the work and quality standards before attempting the time study.

The time study is based upon a fifty minute hour with ten minutes per hour allowed for fatigue and personal breaks. Time study periods should be at least twenty-five minutes in duration. All participants start and end the time study together. Total the number of units completed and subtract the number of units not meeting the quality standard. Divide the total of correct units by the total hours of the participants to determine units per hour. By dividing 3,000 seconds (fifty minutes) by the units per hour you will determine the number of seconds to produce one unit.

EXAMPLE. Twenty-five minute time study.

	Completed	Incorrect
John	12	1
Sue	11	1
Bill	11	2
Total Completed ...	34	4
Incorrect..........	4	
Total Correct	30	

30 Total Correct   1.5 hours = A Rate of 20 units per hour.

SECONDS PER UNIT. 3,000 Sec ÷ 20 units per hour = 150 seconds per unit.

PREPARATION FOR SITUATIONAL ASSESSMENT. The evaluator should then demonstrate the task to the client and insure that he is familiar with the work and quality standards. Each client should practice the task until he can complete it perfectly five consecutive times without error.

Explain to the clients that you will be timing them as they work and they should work as quickly and as carefully as they can.

AT TASK CHARTING WORKSHEET

Task _____

Date _____

Codes

A = At task

A- = At task but not fully attending, i.e. looking up, talking, or ritual behavior

Ax = At task but not fully attending due to organizational distractions, i.e. poor work environment, receiving instructions, or securing supplies

N- = Not at task for same reasons as A-

Nx = Not at task for same organizational reasons as Ax

Minute	Name	Name	Name
1.			
2.			
3.			
4.			
5.			
6.			
7.			
8.			
9.			
10.			
11.			
12.			
13.			
14.			
15.			
16.			
17.			
18.			
19.			
20.			
21.			
22.			
23.			
24.			
25.			
Total A			
A-			
Ax			
N-			
Nx			

Figure 8-1. Courtesy of Robert Morgan, Director of Adult Services, Summit County Board of Mental Retardation, Akron, Ohio.

CONDUCTING THE SITUATIONAL ASSESSMENT. This stage of the assessment is best done with two evaluators. One will observe and note on the Unit Completion Worksheet the time in seconds it takes each evaluee to complete one complete unit. The second evaluator will record each evaluee's behavior at one minute intervals on the At Task Charting Worksheet (see Figure 8-1).

The Unit Completion Worksheet simply records how long it takes the evaluee to complete one work cycle in seconds. The concept of a work cycle is important because it will include any delays incurred before the next unit is started. Each evaluee is sampled in rotation in order to sample the effort at different stages in the work period. Comments on notable problems, inefficiencies or skills are noted next to the recorded time.

During the same work period a second evaluator notes each evaluee's sample behavior on the Task Charting Worksheet. This is done simply by starting every minute and sampling in turn each evaluee's behavior. The sample period for each evaluee should be limited to three to five seconds. The criterion used in the example is only a suggested criterion and it can be adjusted to meet local needs. Additional notes can be made to further clarify the coding or to note special concerns.

The information from both the At Task Charting Worksheet and the Unit Completion Worksheet is then interpreted and transferred to the Individual Performance Record (see Figures 8-2 and 8-3).

The Individual Performance Record provides a format for compiling the results of the timed work period and services as a record to compare performance over a period of time. Once the Individual Performance Records are completed, the worksheets can be discarded.

The total units completed during the twenty-five minute work period are recorded in the first column. Then the number completed not meeting the minimum quality control standards is recorded and subtracted from the total number completed to give the total correct. By then doubling the total correct, we obtain the evaluee's rate per hour. If you divide the rate per hour by the rate from the original time study, it will determine the percentage of rate.

INDIVIDUAL PERFORMANCE RECORD

Workers Name _____ Job Title _____ Normal rate per hour _____

Instructor _____ Job Number _____ Normal rate/sec. per pc. _____

Date _____ Date _____ Date _____

Timed periods	25 min.	60 min.	Timed periods	25 min.	60 min.	Timed periods	25 min.	60 min.
Number done			Number done			Number done		
Number incorrect			Number incorrect			Number incorrect		
Total correct			Total correct			Total correct		
Rate per hour			Rate per hour			Rate per hour		
% of normal rate			% of normal rate			% of normal rate		

Time per piece in second	Range	Average	Time per piece in seconds	Range	Average	Time per piece in seconds	Range	Average

At Task Charting		At Task Charting		At Task Charting	
Code - Count	Notable Behaviors	Code - Count	Notable Behaviors	Code - Count	Notable Behavior
A		A		A	
A-		A-		A-	
Ax		Ax		Ax	
N-		N-		N-	
Nx		Nx		Nx	
Comments and Recommendations		Comments and Recommendations		Comments and Recommendations	

Figure 8-2.

The longest and shortest times to complete a unit are recorded under range and the mean average of the timings is recorded under average.

Charting completed with the At Task Charting Worksheet is totaled by category and recorded next to the appropriate code. Any notable comments or recommendations are also recorded.

At a later time, sample a sixty minute period when the evaluee is working at the same task, but do not indicate that you are measuring his performance. At the end of the sixty minute period, count, inspect, and record his totals (the same as you did for the 25 minute timed study), but do not double the total correct to determine the rate per hour.

Results and Conclusions

What do we look for in all of this information and data to

UNIT COMPLETION WORKSHEET

Date _____   Rate per hour _____

Task _____   Seconds per unit _____

Name	Name	Name
Seconds per Unit	Seconds per Unit	Seconds per Unit
1.	1.	1.
2.	2.	2.
3.	3.	3.
4.	4.	4.
5.	5.	5.
Total	Total	Total
Average – Mean _____	Average – Mean _____	Average – Mean _____
Range High _____	Range High _____	Range High _____
Range Low _____	Range Low _____	Range Low _____
Comments	Comments	Comments
Total Completed _____	Total Completed _____	Total Completed _____
Total Incorrect _____	Total Incorrect _____	Total Incorrect _____
Total Correct _____	Total Correct _____	Total Correct _____

Figure 8-3. Courtesy of Robert Morgan, Director of Adult Services, Summit County Board of Mental Retardation, Akron, Ohio.

better understand the evaluee's potential, habits, strengths, and needs? The following may provide some clues:

1. Workers normally will do the same, or a little better, on the twenty-five minute time work period than they do on the sample work period. If this difference is great, it might indicate the evaluee lets down under less supervision. If the evaluee does better during the sample work period, it may indicate that close supervision or the pressure of the

time period adversely affects his work.

2. A large number of incorrect units, especially during the timed work period, may indicate the client was careless or did not understand the quality standards or could not discriminate the quality control standards.

3. The percent of rate will indicate how the client's performance compares with the non-handicapped individuals who conducted the time study. The sample is not adequate to determine generalized norms, but it does provide some indication as to the client's performance on that task.

4. Variation in range — the longest time it takes to complete one unit compared to the shortest time it takes to complete a similar unit — will indicate the consistency with which the evaluee works.

5. At Task charting will provide not only information about the evaluee's behavior, but also about his environment and how it may affect his work. For example, in one study it was noted that an oscillating fan had caused the evaluee to waste time gathering the work that the fan had blown away. You may also note the effects of other environmental considerations such as lighting problems, noise and visual distractions, bothersome co-workers, and improper stool or table height.

    Non-productive behaviors of the evaluee may also be noted. Examples of non-productive behaviors might include ritualistic movements, over checking of work, inefficient work methods, breaks or pauses between work steps, and visual or verbal attention away from the task.

6. Replication of the study after the task has been practiced will indicate if there has been any improvement with experience.

Situational assessment is a systematic and objective evaluation of how the subject is performing in the actual work site. It can provide the supervisor, teacher, or evaluator with a very accurate view of the variables affecting performance. This information is useful to the evaluee also.

It can help the evaluee have a more realistic view of his/her own abilities and performance. It can help clarify expectations and set goals for the future.

Situational assessment, as the one above, enables us to measure three aspects of the performance:

1. The evaluee's ability to perform the task.
2. The environment's effect on the task.
3. The evaluee's reaction to the environment.

Cartwright and Cartwright (1974) have a detailed discussion of alternative observation techniques that could be applied in a variety of settings and should be of value to the reader.

Task Analysis

Task Analysis is perhaps the most widely used technique of evaluation for the severely multi-handicapped population. The evaluation of the client's performance via task analysis is simply breaking tasks into small discrete steps and noting the client's strengths and weaknesses relative to the components of the specific task. The process of task analysis has been applied to evaluation and training with the severely and multi-handicapped in a variety of settings (Gold, 1976; Karan Wehman, Renzaglia, and Schutz, 1976). Gold (1976; 1978), in the development of his instructional technology, has promoted the term *content task analysis*, which, according to Gold, simply refers to breaking a task into teachable components, with the teachability of the task being determined primarily by the skill of the instructor and the skills of the learner. Gold emphasizes that the most important factor in the process of content task analysis is the necessity of the instructor developing an intense familiarity with the task to be taught. Gold describes the process of task analysis as a somewhat arbitrary or trial and error procedure, i.e. there is no magic procedure involved in conducting a task analysis because the number and complexity of steps needed would vary with the individual. Once rehabilitation professionals get over the idea that there is some mysticism connected with task analysis and realize that through simple hard work and being sensitive to changing functioning of the client, a good task analysis can be accomplished. Gold views three steps as being crucial in the application of the task analysis process: (1) many content task analyses should be prepared and subsequent training attempts implemented: (2) the evaluator/instructor should know the intended population well; and (3) task analyses should be revised frequently (1976).

Gold has developed a very simple procedure for assessing a client's skill level via a content task analysis. As Figure 8-4 illustrates, the procedure merely involves writing each step in the task analysis across the top of a data sheet. The trainer or evaluator simply makes a symbol for a correct, incorrect, or correct-with-assistance response. This strategy allows the evaluator or instructor to become very intimate with the client's performance on a specific task. The alert evaluator could then note areas of difficulty and make revisions so that each trial would result in fewer mistakes being made (Gold, 1978).

The Concept of Work-sample Formats

The use of the work-sample format to evaluate and predict the vocational functioning of various types of handicapped individuals has expanded rapidly in the past ten years. The work-sample format has gained wide use in the evaluation of the work performance of the handicapped because it has been promoted as being superior to standardized assessment instruments by prominent people in the field (Gold, 1973; Neff, 1970; Pruitt, 1970) and by commercial manufacturers of these products.

Neff (1970, p. 27) defines a work-sample as a "mockup, a close simulation of an actual industrial operation, not different in its essentials from the kind of work a potential employer would be required to perform on an ordinary job." Thus, the purpose of the work-sample format is to more closely simulate or approximate the actual job skills (for a specific industrial or workshop setting) the client is being expected to perform. On the surface, this procedure seems to make good sense as the specific vocational skills of interest to the evaluator are being measured much more directly (due to the simulation of a particular industrial or workshop task) than they would be with a "general" standardized procedure such as a pegboard test,

TASK ANALYSIS RECORDING FORM

INDIVIDUAL STEPS — — — — — — — — — — — — — — — — — ➤

	POSTURE	PLACEMENT OF HANDS	GRASP	PICK-UP	ALIGN	INSERT	TURN	TIGHTEN	PUSH
SUCCESSIVE TRIALS 1									
2									
3									
4									
5									
6									
7									

KEY

+ = CORRECT

- = INCORRECT

v = CORRECT WITH ASSISTANCE

Figure 8-4.

which would assess, say, a general category of skills such as fine motor skills. However, certain advantages and disadvantages are inherent in the application of the work-sample strategy in evaluating the work performance of the handicapped. A brief discussion of these advantages and disadvantages is in order.

Advantage of the Work-sample Format:

1. Since the work-sample format simulates a real work situation, the client tends to view the experience as a work task rather than a test, thus providing a "truer" measure of his ability (Hoffman, 1970; Overs, 1968).
2. The work-sample format offers a more controlled setting for the observation of specific work behavior (Neff, 1968).

3. Because they offer a more "real-life" environment, work samples do not tend to be contaminated by such factors as excess anxiety, cultural differences, language problems, cultural differences, and educational level (JEVS, 1968; Neff, 1968; Overs, 1968).
4. Work samples provide the closest approximation of the skills, aptitudes, and abilities required in competitive work environments (JEVS, 1968; Overs, 1968).

Disadvantages of the Work-sample Format:

1. The similarity of the work-sample format to "normal" work tasks can at times be superficial; thus, resemblance in itself does not guarantee a high level of predictive validity (Timmerman and Doctor, 1974; Neff, 1968).
2. The ratings, observations, and interpretations required by the work-sample format, can often only be done subjectively by evaluators (Timmerman and Doctor, 1974).
3. Many work samples have not been adequately validated with the mentally retarded population, and there is a lack of standardization among them (Timmerman and Doctor, 1974).
4. Work samples can be expensive, and their hardware nature complicates the task of periodic revision (Neff, 1968).
5. Because of their lack of rewards for performance, work samples can result in lowering the motivation of the client (Wolfensberger, 1967).

Guidelines and Considerations for Proper Utilization of the Work-Sample Format

Some of the guidelines and considerations for the proper use of work samples are inherent in the listing of advantages/disadvantages; e.g. the practice of simulating an industrial task can, depending upon how carefully it is implemented, be a good or bad procedure.

Certainly, the prudent evaluator would have to take into account the role of motivation in conducting an evaluation via the work-sample format. If the evaluator chooses not to provide for external motivation in having the client undertake a work sample, he should certainly consider this factor in assessing the client's functioning level on a particular task. Thus, criterion failure or a level of performance that the evaluator may feel is below the client's ability level may be due to a considerable extent to a lack of motivation.

The role of training must also be considered in the implementation of the work-sample format. The mentally retarded population has demonstrated a tendency to fail to achieve maximum potential when first being exposed to an unfamiliar task, generally due to a high expectation of failure (Brolin, 1976; Gold, 1973; 1975; Wolfensberger, 1967). Most work samples are designed on the assumption that a strong relationship exists between learning ability and production. Gold (1973; 1975) has rejected this assumption and concludes that contemporary work evaluation procedures frequently result in an underestimation of the work performance level of the mentally retarded population. In commenting on this failure to distinguish between learning ability and production ability, Gold states: "no attempt has been made to make the evaluation period fruitful to the client in terms of the development of the skills which are being evaluated. If anything is gained from the evaluation period, it is usually adjustive in nature with the clients often spending many hours or days being nonproductive and not learning new skills. It is also possible that many retarded clients, who are in a work setting for the first time, develop inappropriate concepts regarding work, which we based on nonproductivity and low level tasks and which are reflected in future performance" (1973, p. 113).

One way to counter this issue of the interaction between acquisition and performance would be tó follow the suggestions of Gold (1973) and Wolfensberger (1967) to reduce the time involved in work evaluation and increase the amount of time the client is engaged in training prior to evaluation. Brolin's (1976) strategy to use a learning curve to graph the client's performance also takes this factor into account. Indeed, the importance of making these modifications is extremely important in the care of the severe and multi-handicapped population.

Finally, as Stodden, Casale, and Schwartz (1977) emphasize, the vocational evaluator must take into account the specific learning and functioning characteristics of the population in question, and include these elements in an overall assessment model. Indeed, a multitude of factors must be considered in order to obtain maximum utility from the evaluation process. For example, there are many interactive factors that have a contribution to successful work performance-employment conditions in the community — values, interests, amount of parental and agency support, and resources for follow-up efforts.

A discussion of some of the more widely used work evaluation systems follows.

Jewish Employment Vocational Service (JEVS)

The JEVS was originally developed to assess the vocational skills of persons who could not speak or write English well enough to take conventional language oriented tests. In the 1960s, under the sponsorship of the United States Department of Labor, the Jewish Employment and Vocational Services in Philadelphia refined the system to assess the work potential of learning disabled, disadvantaged, special needs, and mildly retarded youth and adults.

The system consists of a battery of twenty-eight work samples arranged in a pattern of increasing levels of difficulty in judgment, reasoning, and ability. The twenty-eight samples were selected to minimize the effects of educational deficiencies.

The samples represent ten worker-trait group arrangements of the occupational categories taken from the Dictionary of Occupational Titles — the DOT (United States Department of Labor, 1965; 1966; 1966). Each of the work samples in the ten worker-trait groups relate to data-people-thing hierarchy outlined in the DOT (see McEwen, 1976, for a brief discussion of the DOT data-people-thing hierarchy).

The work samples are administered in a simulated work setting designed to reflect the primary skills inherent in actual jobs. Each work sample is scored in relation to time and quality. The results relate directly to the worker-trait groups in the DOT.

Several criticisms have been made of the JEVS evaluation system. It has been suggested that the client data used to establish norms for time and quality were not adequately researched (Timmerman & Doctor, 1974). The work samples do not adequately reflect the characteristics of the worker trait arrangement group, and some of the worker-trait areas have an insufficient number of items. The institutions for the tasks have been thought to be inadequately matched to the reading and conceptual levels of moderately and mildly retarded individuals (Brolin, 1976; Timmerman & Doctor, 1974). Finally, many evaluators have found that the pressure of time limits the system imposes upon the client can cause undue anxiety and mistakes (Brolin, 1976; Timmerman & Doctor, 1974). The need to disassemble or assemble the work samples so they can be used again is a common criticism of many work-evaluation systems.

JEVS — Vocational Information and Evaluation Work Samples (VIEWS)

Most of the work samples contained in the JEVS system would be too difficult for the moderately/severely retarded and multi-handicapped population. Therefore, the Jewish Employment and Vocational Services developed the VIEWS evaluation system to better assess the work potential of the mentally retarded population. The VIEWS consists of sixteen hands-on work samples representative of worker requirements in occupational areas in which large segments of the American labor force are employed. Like the original JEVS, it is designed to be used in a simulated work environment. The individual samples require no reading skills.

The VIEWS system attempts to account for the role of training. The evaluation process used by the VIEWS consists of a four-stage process:

1. *Orientation* — the client is told about VIEWS, how and why it will be used.
2. *Demonstration* — The client is led through each work sample by the evaluator and is shown the correct procedure to complete each of the tasks.

3. *Training* — The evaluator then trains the client to perform the task until the client masters the activity.
4. *Evaluation* — After the client has achieved the mastery level, he then begins the work sample by himself while the evaluator observes his behavior and scores the sample based upon time and quality.

The VIEWS system, because of this administrative format, has great potential for use with the moderate/severely retarded and multi-handicapped population.

For additional information regarding the JEVS work sample systems write: Jewish Employment and Vocational Services, 1913 Walnut Street, Philadelphia, PA 19103.

McCarrow-Dial Work Evaluation System (MDWES)

The McCarrow-Dial Work Evaluation System (MDWES) is a neurological approach to clinical, vocational, and educational evaluation. Designed to assess the vocational competency and training needs of "mentally disabled" individuals, the MDWES is normed on subgroups of mentally retarded, cerebral-palsied, and severely behaviorally disordered adults from both sheltered workshop and community environments.

The MDWES provides information regarding work potential, suggests appropriate strategies for rehabilitation, and provides information useful in predicting the individual's response potential to an education and rehabilitation program. It is an eclectic approach that incorporates data from other standardized instruments.

The five areas evaluated by the system include the following:

1. *Verbal Cognitive* — depending on the individual client, the protocol and scores are used from the Wechsler Adult Intelligence Scale (WAIS), Wechsler Intelligence Scale for Children — Revised (WISC-R), or Stanford-Binet Intelligence Scale is used. Also, scores from Peabody Picture Vocabulary Test (PPVT), and, for clinical evaluation purposes, results from the Halsted-Reitan Categories Test are often incorporated into the MDWES battery.
   Interview and informal assessment procedures are also

used.
2. *Sensory* — measured by the Bender Visual-Motor Gestalt Test and the Haptec Visual Discrimination Test. Informal techniques for assessing visual-tactual and stereognostic skills often supplement the standardized instrumentation.
3. *Fine and Gross Motor Abilities* — measured by the McCarrow Assessment of Neuromuscular Development (MMAND). In vocational evaluation, the MMAND is often supplemented by specific assessments of range, motion, and physical endurance.
4. *Emotional Adjustment* — measured by the Observational Emotional Inventory. The Minnesota Multi-Phasic Personality Inventory and/or House-Tree-Person drawings are administered when appropriate.
5. *Integration Coping* — measured by the Behavioral Rating Scale and or the Street Survival Skills Questionnaire. These instruments are generally supplemented by interview and behavioral observation.

For additional information on the MDWES, write: Commercial Marketing Enterprises, 11300 North Central Expressway, Suite 105, Royal Central Tower, Dallas, TX 75231.

Singer Vocational Evaluation System

The Singer Vocational Evaluation System consists of a series of work-sample stations that are similar in appearance to study carrels. Each work-sample station contains an audio cassette and filmstrip screen to provide instructions for the task and the necessary tools for the task.

At present, there are seventeen work stations in the Singer system: bench assembly, drafting, basic tools, electrical wiring, plumbing, and pipe fitting, air conditioning and heating, woodwork and carpentry, welding and soldering, clerical, needle trade, medical service, masonry, small engine service, sheet metal work, cooking, cosmetology, and data calculation and recording.

Obviously, some of the work stations in the Singer evaluation system are inappropriate for use with the mentally retarded population. Only a few of the work stations contained in the current Singer evaluation system are considered appropriate for the more severely retarded individual (Stodden, Casale, & Schwartz, 1977). However, the Singer company is currently making efforts to better assess the vocational potential of the moderately and severely retarded population.

As Brolin (1976) indicates, the Singer system has a high degree of face validity and natural appeal due to the elaborate simulation of "real life" work environments. The audio-visual format used in the instruction is a clear advantage in that it provides the client with a more concrete idea of what he is being asked to do. There is an excellent supply of tools to be used in fabricating various products.

Despite its obvious advantage, the Singer evaluation system does seem to have a couple of shortcomings. There is a lack of basic research data to substantiate various features of this system (Brolin, 1976). For example, the procedure and rationale for coordinating the listing of job titles and related DOT numbers to the various work stations is unclear. Some evaluators have been critical of the sound quality of audio instructions and the rather small screen size of the filmstrip screen (personal conversations and experiences of the writers).

For additional information on the Singer evaluation system, write: Singer Educational Division, Career Systems, 80 Commerce Drive, Rochester, NY 14623.

Testing, Orientation, and Work Evaluation in Rehabilitation (TOWER)

The TOWER work-sample format was developed at the ICD Rehabilitation and Research Center in New York City. The TOWER incorporates work tasks covering fourteen areas of work evaluation: clerical, drafting, drawing, electronics assembly, jewelry making, leathergoods, lettering, machine shop, mail clerk, optical mechanics, pantograph, sewing, workshop assembly, and welding.

The total evaluation process with the TOWER system can take as long as three or four weeks as it involves the client in a number of work tasks within an occupational area. The tasks are arranged in a hierarchial fashion so that the last task performed in a specific occupational area will incorporate the use of most of the tools for that area.

The developers claim that the qualitative and quantitative standards for the various sample tasks were established in relation to established industrial requirements. The TOWER protocol is the oldest evaluation system used in rehabilitation settings, having been in use since the early 1940s. It has been used extensively with the mentally retarded and multi-handicapped population. Rosenberg (1967) cites several reasons for the venerability of the TOWER system: the flexible nature of its format, its proven validity; and its closeness in approximating the workshop setting.

Brolin (1976) reports that the flexibility of the TOWER system has resulted in many agencies modifying the various work tasks and standards to adapt to local community vocational opportunities. The reading and comprehension levels of the test instructions in particular have been modified extensively to meet the needs of the mentally retarded.

For more information on the TOWER system, write: ICD Rehabilitation and Research Center, 400 First Avenue, New York, NY 10010.

Valpar Component Work Sample Series

The Valpar Component Work Sample Series is one of the more recent work evaluation systems. It is the result of over ten years of research and development.

The Valpar Component Work Sample Series consists of sixteen independent work samples. Each sample is designed to measure universal worker characteristics found to be the basic indicators of success in numerous job families. This universality of the samples enables facilities to integrate each component with other work samples already in use, thereby enhancing their total vocational evaluation program. The Valpar system is also keyed to the worker trait arrangement data in the DOT. The sixteen samples consist of the following:

1. Small Tool (Mechanical Tasks).
2. Size Discrimination.
3. Numerical Sorting.
4. Upper Extremity Range of Motion.
5. Clerical Comprehension and Aptitude.
6. Independent Problem Solving.
7. Multi-level Sorting.
8. Simulated Assembly.
9. Whole Body Range of Motion.
10. Tri-level Measurement.
11. Eye-Hand-Foot Coordination.
12. Soldering (Electronics).
13. Money Handling.
14. Integrated Peer Performance.
15. Electrical Circuitry and Print Reading.
16. Drafting.

Each sample comes in a self-contained unit with norming data, scoring forms, and an individual work sample manual. Any evaluator who has ever worked with work samples can, after reading the manual, administer the Valpar Component to the client with very little difficulty.

Each sample is normed upon the time of completion, in seconds, and the quality of the performance. In addition, the norm data provided with each sample is broken down into institutionally retarded, shelter living, independent community living, a disadvantaged population, Air Force norms, San Diego employed worker norms, method time measurement norms, deaf norms, and a skill center norm. Each norming population is thoroughly explained in the Valpar Work Sample Component Manual. With the norms supplied in the Valpar Component, the evaluator can match his specific population to a previously-normed population having similar general characteristics. All of the work samples can be normed by the evaluator to his own particular clients if he so chooses.

The Valpar system is unique in that its developers felt that other work samples overlooked the motivational factors involved in completing a work task. Thus, they have tried to develop samples that maximize the client's motivation to complete them.

The multiple norm groups used in the Valpar system are rather limited in scope, thus reducing the validity of comparisons to them. Also, the timing of the work sample in second units reduces the flexibility of the evaluators when dealing with a number of clients simultaneously.

For additional information on the Valpar Component Work Sample System write: Valpar Corporation, 655 North Alvermon Way, Suite 108 Tucson, AZ 85716.

Wide Range Employment Sample Test (WREST)

The WREST is one of the most widely used evaluation systems with the moderately/severely retarded population. This battery was developed by Jastak and King (1972) in a rehabilitation workshop environment. The authors made observations of the most commonly used movements used in typical workshop production situations. The quantitative and qualitative norm data were established with this workshop population. Additional quantitative and qualitative norm data were obtained from populations in regular industry and production situations. The client's readiness to enter the competitive employment market can be assessed by comparison of his performance on the workshop norms to those of the industrial norms.

The WREST consists of a series of ten performance samples, which range in allotted time from one and one-half to fifteen minutes. These ten performance samples are as follows:

1. Single and double folding, pasting, labeling, and stuffing.
2. Stapling.
3. Rice measuring.
4. Screw assembly.
5. Bottle packaging.
6. Pattern making.
7. Color and shade matching.
8. Swatch pasting.
9. Collating.
10. Tag stringing.

The major purpose of the WREST is to assess perceptual and dexterity abilities. The WREST can be administered individually in approximately one and one-half hours.

The performance tasks on the WREST can be repeated as often as desired. The test developers even encourage that the client be taught and coached to help provide an assessment of his ability to perform the tasks when given a valid opportunity. Brolin (1976) views this opportunity to practice the work sample prior to timing as a very advantageous factor for the mentally retarded. This helps the perceptive evaluator to make a judgment of the interaction of the client's acquisition of ability and performance, a factor which, as discussed earlier, should not be overlooked.

Unlike the work evaluation systems discussed earlier, the WREST does not attempt to relate the results of performance on its work samples to the DOT or other classification systems. In reviewing the WREST, Botterbusch (1973) concludes that most of the work samples seemed to correspond closely to the Handling Worker Trait Group (0.887 code, which represents jobs requiring simple materials handling).

Some of the criticisms of the WREST system are that the normative data is limited (Timmerman and Doctor, 1974), the instructions are confusing (Timmerman and Doctor, 1974), and better procedures are needed for observation of client behavior (Brolin, 1976).

Overall, the WREST seems to have significant potential for providing vocationally relevant information for the moderately, severely, and multi-handicapped population.

For additional information on the WREST write: Guidance Associates of Delaware, Inc., 1526 Gilpin Avenue, Wilmington, DL 19806.

APPENDICES

Establishing a Report Form

The following is an example of a reporting form which should maximize the usefulness of the vocational data which has been collected on an individual.

Report Form courtesy of Mr. Ronald Gerstenmaier, Special Needs Evaluation, R. G. Drage Career Education Center, Massillon, Ohio.

APPENDIX A

R. G. DRAGE CAREER EDUCATION CENTER

VOCATIONAL EVALUATION
REPORT FORM

REFERRAL AGENCY_____DATE _9/8/79_____

STUDENT'S NAME__John Smith_____AGE_15___ SEX_M_____

ADDRESS _____SOCIAL SECURITY NO._____

CITY_____STATE_____ ZIP_____

PHONE_____BIRTH DATE _June 24, 1964_____

DATE ENTERED EVALUATION 9/8/79 DATE COMPLETED EVALUATION 9/11/79

DAYS ATTENDED_____4_____   DAYS ABSENT_0_____

CASE #_____

A. Suggested Worker Trait Group Arrangements for employability planning_____

.687 with improvement in speed_____

B. Supportive Services -_____ None __x__Basic Education _____Vocational Counseling

_____ Vocational Training_x_Work-study___Work Adjustment

__x__ Other BVR

C. Significant work characteristics: Pleasant, cooperative, energetic, but work

lacks quality and neatness_____

D. Rationale for Suggestions: Based upon the test scores the test scores and

observations of the vocational evaluator_____

EVALUATOR_____

SUPERVISOR _____

DATE _10/22/79_____

I. *PHYSICAL CHARACTERISTICS*

Grooming, Work Attire, and Physical Description:

Hair __Black__ Eyes __Blue__ Height __5'5"__ Weight __125__

Areas Needing Attention:

__John should be instructed to wear socks with his shoes__

Observed physical problems and the effects upon work performance:_____

II. *COMMUNICATION OBSERVED DURING EVALUATION*

	Satisfactory	Warrants Attention
Speech, Articulation		X
Voice tone	X	
Grammar		X
Conveys thoughts and ideas	X	
Vocabulary development	X	

Explanation of areas needing attention:

__At times the evaluator found it difficult to interpret what John was__

__trying to communicate due to his articulation__

III. *SOCIAL CHARACTERISTICS OBSERVED DURING EVALUATION*

	Satisfactory	Warrants Attention
Personality	X	
Courtesy and manners	X	
Initiates conversations	X	
Participates in conversations	X	
Sense of humor	X	
Eye contact	X	

	Satisfactory	Warrants Attention
Interaction w/male co-worker	___	X
Interaction w/female co-worker	___	X
Cooperation w/supervisors	X	___
Willingly attempts tasks	X	___
Reaction to constructive criticism	X	___
Reaction to praise	X	___
Ability to cooperate with others	X	___
Ability to work alone	X	___
Ability to compete	X	___

Explanation of area needing attention

During the week John exhibited several behaviors which were
inappropriate for his environment.

_____

_____

_____

_____

IV. *INAPPROPRIATE BEHAVIOR OBSERVED DURING EVALUATION*

__X__ None

_____ Withdrawn/Introverted

_____ Overly social to supervisors

_____ Nervous symptoms (stuttering, giggling)

_____ Chronic complaining

_____ Loud, domineering or aggressive

__X__ Other (explain)

_____

_____

_____

_____

V. *WORKER CHARACTERISTICS OBSERVED DURING EVALUATION*

Attendance:

Present __4__ days out of __4__ days

Number of excused absents _____

Punctuality:

__0__ Times late morning arrival

__0___ Times late returning from breaks

__0___ Times late returning from lunch

__0___ Times prepared to leave early

Neatness was observed in the following areas:

_____ Legible handwriting

___X___ Recording numbers legibly

_____ Alignment of numbers

_____ Corrections/erasures

_____ Maintaining work area

_____ Cleaning work area after completion of a sample

___X___ Lack of neatness caused numerous errors

Frustration:

_____ Frequently upset_____X___ Occasionally upset _____Rarely upset

___X___ Ability to control frustration level

_____ Ability to continue inspite of opposition

___X___ Ability to maintain an even temperament

_____ Ability to tolerate pressure

Conditions under which frustration occurred:

__John became frustrated when faced with the Academic and__

__Mechanical tasks of the Evaluation.__

Signs of Frustration:

__Nervousness, distractability, and would ask for further assistance__

__from the evaluator__

Attention Span:

___X___ Adequate

_____ Warrants attention (explanation):

Initative:

___X___ Began on own

_____ Continued on own

___X___ Indicated when ready for next task

___X___ Ability to begin a task without encouragement

_____ Ability to maintain motivation

_____ Ability to concentrate on a task

_____ Ability to make decisions

_____ Ability to believe in or rely on oneself

Planning and organization:

_____ Began by sorting like parts

_____ Arranged tasks in a sequential order

__X___ Over-organized

_____ Changed organization after beginning a task

__X___ Displayed visible signs of a plan for reassembly during disassembly

_____ Conceptualized the problem

_____ Responded to change

_____ Worked haphazardly

_____ Displayed no visible signs of organization

Accuracy:

	Above Average	Average	Below Average
Routine assembly	_____	_____	X
Sorting	X	_____	_____
Routine mechanical	_____	_____	X
Routine clerical	_____	_____	X
Sophisticated mechanical	_____	_____	X
Academic/clerical	_____	_____	X

Speed:

	Above Average	Average	Below Average
Routine assembly	_____	_____	X
Sorting	_____	_____	X
Routine mechanical	_____	_____	X
Routine clerical	_____	_____	X
Sophisticated mechanical	_____	_____	X
Academic/clerical	_____	_____	X

VI. *ACADEMICALLY RELATED COMPETENCIES*

Instructions:

Successfully followed _2_ step verbal instructions

_____ Read written instructions on 5th grade level unassisted

___X___ Followed written directions in a general way

_____ Followed written directions including specific details

_____ Could not or would not attempt to use written directions

_____ Derived general process from diagrammatic instructions

_____ Followed specific details in diagrammatic instructions

___X___ Needed assistance to follow diagrammatic instructions

_____ Visual memory skills

_____ Auditory memory skills

Most effective way to provide instructions:

Verbal_____X_____ Diagrammatic_____ Demonstration__X____

Written _____   Model _____

Numerical skills (with minimum of 75 percent accuracy)

___X___ Counting parts 1-23

___X___ Counting parts 25-100

___X___ Basic addition and subtration

___X___ Multiplication (Hours worked x rate of pay)

_____ Multiplication (Overtime time and one half)

_____ Percentages and decimals

_____ Measuring whole inches under 12"

_____ Measuring fractions in ½ and ¼ of an inch

___X___ Recognition of coins by name

___X___ Recognition of coins by value

___X___ To change coins

___X___ To change paper money

_____ To make change

_____ To apply economic principles

_____ To count money

_____ Measuring fractions in 8ths and 16th of an inch

VII. *DISCRIMINATION*

Sufficient in the areas of:

_____ Form (perceive length, width, detail in graphic materials)

_____ Spatial (visualize two and three dimensional objects)

___X___ Size

___X___ Color

VIII. *MANIPULATIVE SKILLS*

Sufficient in the areas of:

   X   Assembly of large parts

_____ Assembly of small parts

_____ Eye, hand, foot coordination

_____ Eye, hand, finger coordination

_____ Fine motor sufficient for competitive employment

   X   Gross motor sufficient for competitive employment

   X   To maintain physical stamina

   X   To maintain physical stamina for routine assembly work

IX. *BASIC TOOL COMPETENCY*

Use of hand tools used in the evaluation such as screwdrivers, pliers, mallet, tin snips, metal scriber, file, vice, and soldering gun.

_____Proficient   ____X_Satisfactory   _____Unsatisfactory

Recommendations based on the observations made during the vocational evaluation: Based upon the test scores and the observations made during the vocational evaluation. The evaluator recommends that John remain in the special ed class room and receives remediation in: reading for directions, following diagrams, problem solving, measuring whole inches. measuring fractional parts of an inch, multiplying hours work time rate of pay for over time, working with percents and decimals, making change using real money, social behavior, and health and hygiene also a motor activity program to help develop his fine and gross motor skills.

John did not pass any worker train area tested for in the evaluation but did show to have some strength in the .687 worker train area (sorting, inspecting, measuring and related) and could possibly be successfully employed in this area if he could improve his motor skills to the point to where he could become competitive. Work activities in this group primarily involved examining and measuring or weighing objects or materials for the purpose of grading, sorting, detecting flaws or irregularities or verifying a transist of specifications. The work frequently is performed under close supervision and the use of gauges or calipers and other measuring devices or equipment as well as the primary senses are often involved. Workers requirements occupationally sufficient combination of the ability and willingness to follow instructions to the letter spatial and form perception perceive differences in tangible matter. Accuracy and attention to detail, finger and manual dexterity, eye-hand coordination and a disposition toward work of routine repetitive, and non-creative nature.

APPENDIX B

NAME _____John Smith_____ DATE 9/11/79

CASE#_____

SUPPLEMENT TO
VOCATIONAL EDUCATIONAL
REPORT FORM

Work Sample performance is scored on a three point scale with a score of three (3) being the highest and one (1) the lowest. A score of at least two (2) in both time and quality factors must be obtained for the enrollee to be considered as having performed successfully on a Work Sample in any of the Worker Trait Group Arrangements (WTGAs).

Indicated below are the number of work samples to be successfully performed in a WTGA before the enrollee could be considered for occupations within that WTGA. In a WTGA which contains only one Work Sample, consideration must be given to successful performance on Work Samples in other related WTGAs. A circle around the D.O.T. code number indicates successful performance (SP) in that WTGA.

When utilizing the specific Work Sample scores, caution should be given to Work Sample Numbers 10, 11, 12, 20, 30, and 36 which are asterisked and scored only as successfully or unsuccessfully performed. These samples will be scored either 3 (successful performance) or 1 (unsuccessful performance) for quality. Additional information as to the reason for unsuccessful performance is found on the last page of this supplement.

NAME   John Smith   **WORK SAMPLE PERFORMANCE SCORES**

WTGA	CODE	PAGE	WORK SAMPLE		SP	R/T	R/Q
HANDLING	.887	360	1.	Nut, Bolt, & Washer Assembly		1	1
			2.	Rubber Stamping		-	-
Must have SP on 3			3.	Washer Threading		2	1
of 5 Samples			4.	Budgette Assembly		-	-
			5.	Sign Making		3	1
SORTING,	.687	282	*10.	Tile Sorting		1	3
INSPECTING,			*11.	Nut Packing		1	3
MEASURING			*12.	Collating Leather Samples		-	-
AND RELATED							
Must have SP on 2							
of 3 Samples							
TENDING	.885	447	*20.	Grommet Assembly		1	3
Must also have SP							
in Handling &/or							
Sorting Insp., Meas.							
WTGA and on any							
2 Manipulating							
MANIPULATING	.884	322	*30.	Union Assembly		1	1
			31.	Belt Assembly		3	1
			32.	Ladder Assembly		-	-
Must have SP in 4			33.	Metal Square Fabrication		1	1
of 7 Samples			34.	Hardware Assembly		-	-
			35.	Telephone Assembly		2	1
			*36.	Lock Assembly			
ROUTINE	.688	289	40.	Filing by Numbers			
CHECKING &			41.	Proofreading		-	-
RECORDING							
Must have SP on							
both Samples							
CLASSIFYING,	.388	276	50.	Filing by Letters		-	-
FILING &			51.	Nail & Screw Sorting		1	1
RELATED			52.	Adding Machine		1	1
Must have SP on			53.	Payroll Computation		1	1
3 of 5 Samples			54.	Computing Postage		-	-
INSPECTING &	.487	271	60.	Resistor Reading		-	-
STOCK CHECK-							
ING							
Must also have SP							
on #53 and #54							
CRAFTSMAN-	.381	312	70.	Pipe Assembly		-	-
SHIP & RE-							
LATED							
Must also have SP							
on #60, or #80, or							
#80a, or #90							
COSTUMING,	.361	308	80.	Blouse Making		-	-
TAILORING &			80a.	Vest Making		-	-
DRESSMAKING							
Must also have SP							
on #60 or #70							
DRAFTING AND	.281	377	90.	Condensing Principle		-	-
RELATED							
Must also have SP							
on #60, or #70, or							
#80, or #80a.							

NAME_____John Smith_____

WORK SAMPLE NUMBER AND NAME	REASON(s) FOR UNSUCCESSFUL PERFORMANCE
#10 Tile Sorting	Client took over allotted time for completion
#11 Nut Packing	Same
#12 Collating Leather Samples	
#20 Grommet Assembly	Same
#30 Union Assembly	Client was unable to duplicate the diagram
#36 Lock Assembly	Client was unable to reassemble after disassembly

APPENDIX C

VALPAR Component Work Sample Score Sheet

No.	Sample	Worker Trait Groups	Rate Time	Rate Quality	Success Performed
#1	Small Tools (Mechanical)	.281 .381 .780 .781 .884	65 45	95 95	79 52
#2	Size Discrimination	.884 .781			
#3	Numerical Sorting	.484 .485 .584 .587 .588 .684 .685 .687 .688			
#4	Upper Extremity Motion (Physical Demands)	Dot Volume 11 pp. 654-656, Demands 4 & 6			
#5	Clerical Comprehension and Aptitude Part A (General Clerical)	.138 .268 .288 .368 .388 .468 .588 .862 .878			
	Part B (Bookkeeping)				
	Part C (Typing)				
#6	Independent Problem Solving	.138 .368 .388 .488 .588 .648 .688 .887 .884			
#7	Multi-Level Sorting	.281 .283 .381 .382 .383 .483 .884	25	70	36
#8	Simulated Assembly	.885 .886 .887	10	10	10
#9	Whole Body Range of Motion (physical Demands)	Dot Volume 11 pp. 654-656, Demands 3-4-6			
#10	Tri-Level Measurement	.280 .281 .381 .687 .781 .782 .884 .885 .886			
#11	Eye-Hand-Foot Coordination	.281 .380 .381 .782 .883 .885 .887	75	20	41
#12	Soldering and Inspecting (Electronic)	.281 .781 .884			
#13	Money - Handling Part A Basic Economics	.168 .268 .288 .368 .388 .468 .478 .488	-5	-5	-5
	Part B Change Making				
	Part C Applied Economics	.			
#14	Integrated Peer Performance	Dot Volume 11 pp. 653-655,11 Aptitudes K,F,M, C,IV Temperaments 1,2, 3,4,5,8 and 9, Physical Demands 4,5 and 6			
#15	Electrical Circuitry and Print Reading	.281 .381 .884 .678			
#16	Drafting B. Measuring	.281 .188 .188			
	C. Line Perception				
	D. Use of Ruler, T-Square and Triangle				
	E. Use of Compass and Circle Template				
	F. Blueprint Reading				
	G. Orthographic Projection				

REFERENCES

Allen, C., and Skinnick, M. Placement through a job trial approach to vocational evaluation. *Vocational Evaluation and Work Adjustment Bulletin, 6 (4)*: 29-33, 1973.

Becker, R. L., and Ferguson, R. E. A vocational picture interest inventory for educable retarded youth. *Except Child, 35*: 562-63, 1969, (b).

Becker, R. L., and Ferguson, R. E. Assessing educable retardates' vocational interests through a non-reading technique. *Ment Retard, 1*: 20-25, 1969, (a).

Becker, W. C. *An Empirical Basis for Change in Education.* Chicago: Sci Res, 1971.

Becker, W., and Engelmann, S. Systems for basic instruction: theory and application. In T. A. Brigham and A. C. Catania (Eds.): *Applied Behavioral Research.* New York: Wiley, 1977.

Becker, W., Engelmann, S., and Thomas, D. *Teaching: A Course in Applied Psychology.* Chicago: Sci Res, 1971.

Becker, W., Engelmann, S., and Thomas, D. *Teaching 2: Cognitive Learning and Instruction.* Chicago: Sci Res, 1975.

Bellamy, G. T., Peterson, L., and Close, D. Habilitation of severely and profoundly retarded: illustrations of competence. *Education and Training of the Mentally Retarded, 10*: 174-186, 1975.

Bijou, S. W. A functional analysis of retarded development. In N. R. Ellis (Ed.): *International Review of Research in Mental Retardation,* vol. 1. New York: Acad Pr, 1966.

Bitter, J. A., and Bolanovich, D. J. Warf: A scale for measuring job-readiness behaviors. *Am J Ment Defic, 74*: 616-621, 1970.

Bitter, J. Bias effect on validity and reliability of a rating scale. *Measurement and Evaluation in Guidance, 3 (2)*: 70-75, 1970.

Bitter, J. Using employer job-sites in evaluation of the mentally retarded for employability. *Ment Retard, 5 (3)*: 21-22, 1967.

Botterbrisch, K. F. Wide range employment sample test. *Vocational Evaluation and Work Adjustment Bulletin, 6 (2)*: 40-43, 1973.

Brolin, D. E. *Vocational Preparation of Retarded Citizens.* Columbus, Ohio: Merrill, 1976.

Buros, O. K. (Ed.): *The Seventh Mental Measurements Yearbook* (2 vols.). Highland Park, N.J.: Gryphon Pr, 1972.

Cartwright, C. A., & Cartwright, G. P. *Developing Observational Skills.* New York: McGraw, 1974.

Dictionary of Occupational Titles, United States Department of Labor, United States Employment Service, Washington, D.C., U.S. Govt. Print. Office, 1965.

Flexer, R. W., and Martin, A. S. Sheltered workshops and vocational training settings. In M. E. Snell (Ed.): *Systematic Instruction of the Moderately and Severely Handicapped.* Columbus, Ohio: Merrill, 1978.

Gillman, W. Adapting the rehabilitation workshop to the needs of the disadvantaged. In W. H. Button (Ed.): *Rehabilitation, Sheltered*

Workshops, and the Disadvantaged: An Exploration in Manpower Policy. Ithaca, N.Y.: Cornell U Pr, 1970.

Gold, M. W., and Pomerantz, D. J. Issues in prevocational training. In M. E. Snell (Ed.): *Systematic Instruction of the Moderately and Severely Handicapped.* Columbus, Ohio: Merrill, 1978.

Gold, M. W. Research on the vocational habilitation of the handicapped: the present, the future. In N. R. Ellis (Ed.): *International Review of Research in Mental Retardation,* vol. 6. New York: Acad Pr, 1973.

Gold, M. W. Stimulus factors in skill training of retarded adolescents on a complex assembly task: acquisition, transfer, and retention. *Am J Ment Defic, 76:* 517-526, 1972.

Gold, M. W. Task analysis of a complex assembly task by the retarded blind. *Except Child, 42:* 78-84, 1976.

Gold, M. W. Vocational training. In J. Wortis (Ed.): *Mental Retardation and Developmental Disabilities: An Annual Review,* vol. 7. New York: Brunner-Mazel, 1975.

Hoffman, P. R. An overview of work evaluation. *J Rehabil, 36 (1):* 16-18, 1970.

Homer, R. H., and Bellamy, G. T. A conceptual analysis of vocational training. In M. E. Snell (Ed.): *Systematic Instruction of the Moderately and Severely Handicapped.* Columbus, Ohio: Merrill, 1978.

Huddle, D. Work performance of trainable adults as influenced by competition, cooperation, and monetary reward. *Am J Ment Defic, 72:* 198-211, 1967.

Hunter, J., and Bellamy, G. T. Cable harness construction for severely retarded adults: a demonstration of training technique. *AAESPH Review, 1 (7):* 2-13, 1976.

Jens, K., and Shores, R. Behavioral graphs as reinforcers for work behavior of mentally retarded adolescents. *Education and Training of the Mentally Retarded, 4:* 21-26, 1969.

Jewish Employment and Vocational Service. *Work-sample Program Experimental and Demonstration Project.* Philadelphia: Jewish Employment and Vocational Service, 1968.

Karan, O., Wehman, P., Renzaglia, A., and Schultz, R. *Habilitation Practices with the Severely Developmentally Disabled,* vol. 1. Madison, WI: Research and Training Center in Mental Retardation, University of Wisconsin, Madison, 1976.

Lustig, P. Differential use of the work situation in the sheltered workshop. *Rehabil Lit, 31 (2):* 39-42, 49, 1970.

Martin, A. W., and Morris, J. L. *Development of a General Purpose Vocational Assessment Technique* Annual Progress Report. Lubbock, Texas: Research and Training Center in Mental Retardation, 1977.

Matey, C. *Guidelines for Assessment of Low Incidence Handicapped and Multiimpaired Children.* Dayton, Ohio: The Miami Valley Regional Center for Handicapped Children, 1975.

McEwen, M. L. Career guidance and the dictionary of occupational titles.

Except Child, 42 (10): 31-33, 1976.

Merachnik, D. Assessing work potential of the handicapped in public school. *Vocational Guidance Quarterly, 18 (3):* 225-229, 1970.

Nadolsky, J. Evaluation criteria: an essential precessor to systematic vocational evaluation. *Rehabilitation Counseling Bulletin, 9 (3):* 89-94, 1966.

Nadolsky, J. Patterns of consistency among vocational evaluators. *Vocational Evaluation and Work Adjustment Bulletin, 4 (4):* 13-25, 1971.

Neff, W. S. Problems of work evaluation. *Personnel and Guidance Journal, 24:* 682-688, 1966.

Neff, W. Vocational assessment theory and models. *J Rehabil, 36 (1):* 27-29, 1970.

Neff, W. *Work and Human Behavior.* New York: Aldine-Atherton, 1968.

Overs, R. *The Theory of Job Sample Tasks.* Milwaukee: Curative Workshop, 1968.

Overs, R. Vocational evaluation: research and implications. *J Rehabil, 36 (1):* 18-21, 1970.

Paulsen, A. *The VIEWS System: A Source of Objective Information on Vocational Potential of the Mentally Retarded.* Philadelphia: Jewish Employment and Vocational Service, 1978.

Peterson, R., and Jones, E. M. *Guide to Jobs for the Mentally Retarded.* Pittsburgh: Am Inst Res, 1964.

Pomerantz, D., and Marholin, D. Vocational habilitation: A time for change. In E. Sontag (Ed.): *Educational Programming of the Severely and Profoundly Handicapped.* Reston, VA: Council for Exceptional Children, 1977.

Pruitt, W. Basic assumptions underlying work sample theory. *J Rehabil, 36 (1):* 24-26, 1970.

Rogers, H. B. Time study. In M. M. Dolnick (Ed.): *Contract Procurement Practices of Sheltered Workshops.* Washington, D.C.: U.S. Govt. Print. Office, 1963.

Rosenberg, B. The job sample in vocational evaluation. *Final Report.* New York: Institute for the Crippled and Disabled, 1967.

Salvia, J., & Yneldyke, J. E. *Assessment in Special and Remedial Education.* Boston: Houghton-Mifflin, 1978.

Screven, C., Straka, J., and LaFond, R. Applied behavioral technology in a vocational rehabilitation setting. In W. Gardner (Ed.): *Behavior Modification in Mental Retardation.* Chicago: Aldine, 1971.

Sontag, E. (Ed.). *Educational programming for the severely and profoundly handicapped.* Reston, VA: Council for Exceptional Children, 1977.

Stodden, R. A., Casale, J., and Schwartz, S. E. Work evaluation and the mentally retarded: Review and recommendations. *Ment Retard, 15 (4):* 24-27, 1977.

Thunder, S. K. *The Use of the J.E.V.S. Work Evaluation System With a Handicapped High School Population.* Paper presented at the American Vocational Association Convention, New Orleans, LA,

December 7, 1974.

Timmerman, W. J., and Doctor, A. C. *Special Applications of Work Evaluation Techniques for Prediction of Employability of the Trainable Mentally Retarded.* Stiyker, OH: Quadro Rehabilitation Center, 1974.

U.S. Department of Health, Education, and Welfare. *Placement and Followup in the Vocational Rehabilitation Process.* Washington, D.C.: Ninth Institute on Rehabilitation Services, 1971.

U.S. Government Printing Office. Standards for rehabilitation facilities and sheltered workshops (U.S. Department of Health, Education, and Welfare, Publication No. (SRS) 72-25010, Div. Ed.). Washington, D.C.: Author, 1971.

Walls, R. T., Werner, T. J., Bacon, A., and Zane, T. Behavior checklists. In R. P. Hawkins and J. D. Cone (Eds.): *Behavioral Assessment: New Directions in Clinical Psychology.* New York: Brunner-Mazel, 1977.

Walls, R. T., and Werner, T. J. Vocational behavior checklists. *Ment Retard, 15 (4)*: 30-35, 1977.

Wolfensbergh, W. Vocational preparation and occupation. In A. A. Baumeister (Ed.): *Mental Retardation: Appraisal, Education, and Rehabilitation.* Chicago: Aldine, 1967.

Zimmerman, J., Stuckey, T., Garlick, B., and Miller, M. Effects of token reinforcement on productivity in multiply handicapped clients in a sheltered workshop. *Rehabil Lit, 30*: 34-41, 1969.

U.S. Department of Labor. *Dictionary of Occupational Titles* (3 vols.). Washington, D.C.: U.S. Govt. Print. Office, 1965, 1966, 1966.

BEHAVIOR CHECKLIST REFERENCES

AAMD Adaptive Behavior Scale (1974 revision). American Association of Mental Deficiency, 5201 Connecticut Avenue, N.W., Washington, D.C. 20015.

Behavioral Characteristics Progression. VORT Corporation, P. O. Box 11132, Palo Alto, CA 94306.

Camelot Behavioral Checklists. (Ray W. Foster) Camelot Behavioral Systems, P. O. Box 607, Parsons, KS 67357.

Colorado Master Planning Guide for Instructional Objectives, Division of Developmental Disabilities, 4150 South Lowell, Denver, CO 80236.

COMPET: Commonwealth Plan for Education and Training of Mentally Retarded Children (Pennsylvania Department of Education). Department of Education, Box 911, Harrisburg, PA 17120.

Group Home Candidate Checklist. (Ann P. Turnbull). Department of Special Education, University of North Carolina, Chapel Hill, N.C. 27514

Household Activities Performance Evaluation (William R. Phelps). Disabled Homemaker Program, Division of Vocational Rehabilitation, Charleston, WV 25305.

Jastak-King Work Samples Manual. Wilmington, Delaware: Guidance Associates of Delaware, 1972.

Jewish Employment and Vocational Service. Work-sample program experimental & demonstration project. Philadelphia: Jewish Employment and Vocational Service, 1968.

Job-Seeking Skills Reference Manual. Multi-Resource Centers, Inc., 1900 Chicago Avenue, Minneapolis, MN 55404.

Life Skills for the Developmentally Disabled, Vol. III. (Geneva Folsom) George Washington University, Division of Rehabilitation Medicine, 2300 Eye Street, N.W., Washington, D.C. 20037.

Materials Development Center Behavior Identification Form. Materials Development Center, Department of Rehabilitation and Manpower Services, University of Wisconsin — Stout, Menomonie, WI 54751.

Mid-Nebraska Competitive Employment Screening Test and Teaching Manual. (Robert L. Schalock). Mid-Nebraska Mental Retardation Services, 518 East Side Boulevard, Hastings, NE 68901.

Scale of Employability. Research Utilization Laboratory, Jewish Vocational Service, One South Franklin Street, Chicago, IL 60606.

Social Prevocational Information Battery (SPIB). CTBI McGraw-Hill, Del Monte Research Park, Monterey, CA 93940.

TMR Performance Profile for the Severely and Moderately Retarded. (Alfred J. DiNola, Bernard P. Kaminsky, and Allan E. Sternfield). Educational Performance Associates, 563 Westview Avenue, Ridgefield, NJ 07657.

Vineland Social Maturity Scale. (Edgar Doll). American Guidance Service, Inc., Publisher's Building, Circle Pines, MN 55014.

Vocational Information and Evaluation Work Sample (VIEWS). (Jewish Employment and Vocational Service). Philadelphia: Vocational Research Institute, 1976.

W. A. Howe, Development Center Behavioral Checklist. W. A. Howe Developmental Center, 7600 W. 183rd Street, Tinley Park, IL 60477.

Work Behavior Rating Scale. Exceptional Children's Foundation, 2225 West Adams Boulevard, Los Angeles, CA 90018.

CHAPTER NINE

ASSESSMENT AND THE INDIVIDUALIZED EDUCATIONAL PLAN (IEP): IMPLEMENTING ASSESSMENT DATA

Elizabeth Murray, M.Ed.

THROUGHOUT all of the preceding chapters of this book, emphasis has been placed on obtaining the most comprehensive, unbiased, and accurate evaluation of the multi-handicapped youngster as is possible. This emphasis now shifts to using the accumulated data to provide assistance in the preparation, implementation, and evaluation of individualized programs based on the identified needs, strengths, and weaknesses of the children assessed.

For too long, psychoeducational evaluations served primarily as vehicles for identifying children eligible for special class placement, with the information gathered being frequently irrelevant, insufficient, or even unintelligible to those responsible for determining the child's educational program. The first section of this chapter will investigate how the use of assessment data has changed due to the mandates of Public Law 94-142, suggesting ways in which the assessment team can provide meaningful data to those persons responsible for developing an Individualized Educational Plan (IEP) designed specifically for the child.

Because assessment plays so vital a role in the IEP process, emphasis will next shift to an in-depth review of the contents of the IEP, selection of participants who serve on the IEP team, and the responsibilities of various parties in the IEP process. A thorough understanding of this information is the responsibility of those involved in the assessment, since they will be called upon to serve as active participants in the formation of the IEP document which will determine the child's educational program.

Through the use of a question and answer format, the chapter will conclude with miscellaneous concerns related to the assessment and placement of handicapped children.

THE USE OF ASSESSMENT DATA

Following completion of the Multi-Factored Assessment (MFE), the major task facing the evaluators is one of compiling the data in an organized fashion so that the information can be presented to the IEP team in a clear and concise manner. This section will focus on the process by which the information is passed from the assessment team to the planners of the IEP, suggesting ways in which the data can be most effectively conveyed.

What is the Purpose of the Evaluation Report?

Any time an evaluation is conducted for the purpose of determining whether special education programming or services may be required, the rationale of all assessment efforts should focus on two major goals: (1) determining whether a handicapping condition does, indeed, exist; and (2) furnishing the IEP team members with relevant data which will assist in the determination of appropriate educational programs and services geared to the special needs of the student.

Until the advent of P.L. 94-142, evaluation concentrated almost exclusively on the first of these purposes, i.e. determining eligibility for special education, with the assessment team (or, more frequently, the psychologist) concluding its responsibility with the decision to place or not to place. Students were frequently assigned to special programs on the basis of descriptive data, and consequently, no information concerning the child's educational needs was provided. While the importance of determining whether, indeed, the child is handicapped remains undiminished, the present emphasis of providing information pertinent to educational planning has become one of equal or greater importance.

This increase in the demands made upon the assessment team obviously affects the contents of the evaluation and subsequent report, since the information conveyed now serves as the primary source upon which programming decisions are based. The importance of a relevant, functional, clearly understood assessment report can not therefore be overemphasized, since the effectiveness of educational decisions is clearly based on its contents.

How Does Assessment Fit Into the Mandates of P.L. 94-142?

In order to insure that each youngster considered for special education programming and/or services receives an unbiased, comprehensive, and functional evaluation, P.L. 94-142 mandates that:

1. The instruments and procedures used must be unbiased (121a.531).
2. Whenever possible, the evaluation must be conducted in the child's native language (121a.532al).
3. The instruments used must be employed for the purposes intended by their writers (121a.532a2).
4. The evaluation must be conducted by trained personnel (121a.532a3).
5. A test battery consisting of more than an intelligence test must be employed (121a.532b).
6. Test instruments must be employed which measure aptitude or achievement, not merely reflect impairments (121a.532c).
7. A variety of procedures must be employed (121a.532c).
8. A multidisciplinary team must conduct the evaluation (121a.532e).
9. The evaluation must be comprehensive, addressing all areas related to the suspected disability (121a.532f).

Addressing the procedural safeguards for evaluation, P.L. 94-142 requires that:

1. No individual evaluation may be conducted until the parent consents in writing to the evaluation, having been informed in his native language of all information relevant to the evaluation, including that consent is voluntary

and may be withdrawn at any time, the uses to which the information gathered will be employed, and who will have access to the records (121a.500).

2. The individual evaluation must be conducted prior to any placement in special education programs (121a.531).
3. Children receiving special education services must be re-evaluated with a multifactored battery of instruments at least once every three years, and more frequently if requested by the parents or teacher (121a.534).

P.L. 94-142 also specifies how the assessment data is to be used by the IEP team. It mandates that:

1. Information from a variety of sources must be considered, including achievement and aptitude data, teacher recommendations, social and cultural background information, and measures of adaptive behavior (121a.533al).
2. The data must be documented (121a.533a2).
3. Persons knowledgable in the meaning of the evaluation data and placement options must be involved in the IEP meetings (121a.533a3).

(Note: See Chapter One for more discussion of these legalities).

Where Does Assessment Fit Into the Scheme of Special Education?

The process by which a child receives special education services can be broken into five overlapping stages. These are:

1. the identification of a suspected disability and referral for evaluation;
2. assessment;
3. planning an intervention program based on the child's identified needs (IEP planning);
4. implementation of the special education programming determined in Stage Three; and
5. reviewing and revising the intervention plan on at least an annual basis.

This process can be roughly depicted pictorially (see Figure

9-1). Following the identification of a youngster suspected of having one or more handicapping conditions which may be aided by special education intervention, a formal referral is made. A conference is then held with the parents to explain the assessment process and their due process rights and to obtain their written approval for the evaluation to proceed. Assessment personnel may or may not be involved in this pre-evaluation conference, the important factor being that someone well versed in local procedures and state and federal guidelines chair the meeting.

The process next moves into Stage Two, at which time the formal assessment, including classroom observations, input from teachers, parents, and the child himself, medical evaluation (if necessary), as well as diagnostic and prescriptive assessment, is conducted. This information is consolidated into an assessment report which is then shared with the members of the IEP team to determine the most appropriate placement for the child. Should a youngster qualify for special education placement and/or services, the procedure moves on to Stage Three. The process ends here for those children not found to require special intervention.

An IEP conference is then held in which the child's individualized plan is determined and written. Once more, parental involvement is required, as input from the parents should help determine priorities in the intervention strategies and goals. The parent's signature is required on the IEP document as a means of ensuring that they are aware of their child's plan. Only after these first three stages are completed can a child be served in special education programs.

The child's educational plan forms the basis upon which Stage Four is implemented, as the special programs and/or services determined to be appropriate are provided. This stage lasts only as long as indicated on the IEP, and while many youngsters may require special intervention throughout their school years, a particular implementation plan serves to determine educational intervention for a maximum of one school year, at which time Stage Five — determining the appropriateness of present intervention — is entered. This ensures that no youngster will be placed in special education and forgotten, but

FIGURE 9-1: THE SPECIAL EDUCATION PROCESS

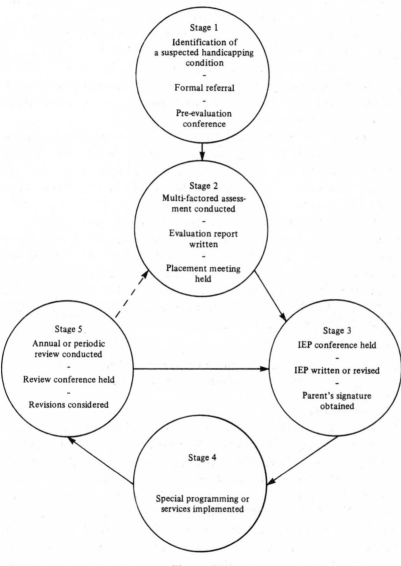

Figure 9-1.

will be given individual attention on at least an annual basis. Under normal circumstances the special education process then focuses only on Stages Three, Four, and Five, as the handicapped child receives special services with a revised IEP being developed on at least an annual basis, thus ensuring that the appropriateness of the intervention be considered periodically. Every third year (or more frequently, if desired), Stage Two again becomes involved so that each identified handicapped child can be re-evaluated to determine whether special education is still warranted and/or whether new strengths and weaknesses should be considered in planning future individualized educational programs.

It should be emphasized that this is a continuous process where the major thrust of the evaluation lies in the Second Stage, in which the assessment team conducts the formal appraisal. Assessment also plays a major role in the Fifth Stage, when the implementation program is reviewed. This provides an important accountability measure for special education intervention. Evaluation should not be considered a discrete event, however, as ongoing appraisal takes place whenever knowledge of the child expands, intervention techniques are found effective or ineffective, or events in the child's personal "sphere," (i.e. birth or death in the family, moving, a new hobby or interest) intervene.

What Types of Information Should the Assessment Team Provide?

As previously stated, assessment serves two major purposes: determining whether a handicapping condition is present which requires special education programming and/or services; and reporting data which will assist in educational planning. As such, the information provided to the IEP team should include *descriptive* data necessary for making placement decisions (WRAT, WISC-R, or Bender results being examples) as well as *prescriptive* data which provides practical information pertinent to program development (this is usually provided through criterion-referenced or competency-based performance measures, classroom observation, and data provided by teachers, parents, or the child).

More specifically, the IEP team will need the following types of information:

1. data describing the child's present level of educational performance;
2. some indication of how the youngster can perform in various educational settings or under specific conditions (i.e. small group vs. large group instruction, structured vs. unstructured settings, auditory vs. visual learning);
3. recommendations concerning what goals and objectives would be appropriate for the child, as well as special techniques or materials which might assist in the child's education; and
4. results of tests used for determination of eligibility (as required by P.L. 94-142), with specific comments regarding the degree of confidence held in these results.

Since the information may be used by persons lacking sophistication in the terminology of assessment, technical jargon should be avoided and the information presented in a clear, understandable manner. Care should also be taken not to "prescribe" treatment in the assessment report, since this is the job of the IEP team. Additionally, only information pertinent to placement eligibility and/or programming needs should be included in the report, and every effort should be made to present the data in as objective a manner as possible.

How Should Assessment Information be Relayed?

Traditionally, each person participating in the assessment process completed his/her evaluation and presented the findings to the IEP team. While this procedure is still practiced in many areas, there are a number of drawbacks to this system, including a great possibility of duplication of effort, inefficiency in terms of time, and the possibility that the IEP team will become so cumbersome as to slow down progress.

An alternative procedure presently being employed in an increasing number of school districts is one of forming an assessment team, which meets prior to the IEP conferences, to consolidate their findings into one comprehensive report so that this single, coherent document can be presented to the IEP team by one representative of the assessment team.

Synthesis of accumulated data may be accomplished by using a common format in which each assessor can relay test data, observations, and anecdotal information under such major headings as Educational Performance, Social/Emotional Development, Cognitive Functioning, and Physical Development. These reports can then be consolidated into one relevant, brief, and understandable document in which present level of functioning and the child's performance under various conditions can be highlighted.

Since those persons responsible for conducting the assessment play so vital a role in the IEP process, and since the information they provide forms the basis upon which all educational decisions are made, this chapter will now turn to an in-depth examination of the IEP, focusing on the components and participants as well as the responsibilities of the local school district in the IEP process.

IEP: THE CONTENT

Following the identification of handicapped students via the "Multi-Factored Assessment" (MFE) discussed in the previous chapters, an "Individualized Education Program" (IEP) must be implemented for each student who is receiving or will receive special services. Responsibility for such plans falls on the local educational agency, with the state educational agency assuming the responsibility of monitoring the compliance of the locally developed plan with the state's guidelines.

While no national movement is underway to develop a uniform format for this written document, a series of guidelines designed to assist in the development of the IEP is provided in P.L. 94-142. Specifically, the law mandates that the IEP must include:

1. a statement of the child's present levels of educational performance;
2. a statement of annual goals, including short-term instructional objectives;
3. a statement of the specific special education and related services to be provided to the child, and the extent to

which the child will be able to participate in regular education programs;

4. the projected dates for initiation of services and the anticipated duration of the services; and

5. appropriate objective criteria and evaluation procedures and schedules for determining, on at least an annual basis, whether the short-term instructional objectives are being achieved.

(Section 121a.346 of Title 45, Public Welfare)

Consideration of each requirement is deemed appropriate, since these describe the minimum information necessary in order to develop IEPs which are in compliance with the federal mandates.

1. A STATEMENT OF THE CHILD'S PRESENT LEVELS OF EDUCATIONAL PERFORMANCE. Data included in this section of the IEP should be based on the results of the MFE and should provide information regarding the student's present functioning in such areas as social and emotional adjustment, vocational and prevocational skills, communication skills, academic achievement, cognitive ability, and daily living skills.

Guidelines for determining what data should be included differs from location to location, with some systems insisting that all psychoeducational data used to determine eligibility for special education be included on the IEP (including IQ scores). More frequently, however, data pertinent to the special programming needs of the student is all that is included in this section. The major emphasis, regardless of local criteria, should be provision of data, indicating the areas that will be emphasized in the special education services/programming of the child, stated in functional terms, and meaningful to the parents, teachers, and students affected by the plan.

2. A STATEMENT OF ANNUAL GOALS, INCLUDING SHORT-TERM INSTRUCTIONAL OBJECTIVES. Information describing what the child can and cannot do, as provided in the statement of present level of educational performance, forms the basis upon which annual goals should be determined. The major challenge in selecting these goals, which should be indicators of what progress is expected within one calendar year, is deter-

mining what the student should learn next.

The identification of these needs might best be accomplished by comparing the current functional status of the youngster with the corresponding desired state of affairs, evaluating the discrepancy between these two, then establishing priorities for intervention which will lead directly or indirectly toward independent functioning. While all areas of need might not be addressed during any one year, it is expected that each will receive attention at some time during the student's educational experience.

For each annual goal, one or more short-term instructional objectives, defined as discrete intermediate steps toward the accomplishment of the stated annual goals, must be identified. These short-term objectives should be specific and concrete and should be behaviorally written and measurable, since they will form the objective basis upon which the IEP can be evaluated. Identification of short-term instructional objectives is best accomplished by considering the steps needed to reach the annual goal, then selecting several of these steps which serve as milestones towards its accomplishment.

The most popular method of presenting the required information is individually writing goals in global terms, i.e. the child will be able to identify the basic colors, and short-term objectives in behavioral terms, i.e. the child will be able to correctly select color tiles as directed by the teacher. Another approach is to develop standardized checklists upon which pertinent goals and objectives can be highlighted. A copy can then be attached to the IEP form.

3. A STATEMENT OF THE SPECIFIC SPECIAL EDUCATION AND RELATED SERVICES TO BE PROVIDED TO THE CHILD, AND THE EXTENT TO WHICH THE CHILD WILL BE ABLE TO PARTICIPATE IN REGULAR EDUCATIONAL PROGRAMS. Information gathered through the MFE, observation of the student, and input from parents, teachers, and the child contribute to the determination of the specific special education and related service needs of the handicapped youngster. Identified needs, including special materials, are to be indicated on the IEP. While not mandatory, most formats also provide space to indicate the percentage of time the child will spend receiving each service. It is the respon-

sibility of the local educational agency to provide any programs or services listed on the IEP. With this in mind, a careful examination of the programs available within the school district should be undertaken. In addition, one should understand the special services/programs in neighboring districts which will provide assistance to students so that realistic program and related service provisions can be made.

Typically, the multi-handicapped youngster requires a variety of special programs, ranging from occupational and/or physical therapy to counseling or psychological services. Regardless of the number of special programs involved, only one IEP is prepared per child, necessitating a team approach to the development and implementation of the document.

Transportation, hydrotherapy, speech pathology, audiology, psychological services, recreation, and occupational therapy are examples of "related services" frequently included on the IEP, although these may be routine parts of some special education programs. The federal regulations make it clear that physical education services must be made available to every handicapped child, even if this requires adaptive programming specifically designed for the youngster. School health services must also be provided, even for students on home instruction.

The second phase of this mandate states that the extent to which the child will be able to participate in regular education programs must be addressed. This is the provision that insures the "least restrictive environment" be considered, since every effort must be made to allow the student the opportunity to participate in regular academic, nonacademic, and extracurricular activities to the maximum extent possible.

While the extent of participation with nonhandicapped students must be indicated on the IEP, annual goals and short-term instructional objectives do not need to be included in areas not provided for by special education or related services. Deciding which areas should be included or, indeed, deciding whether an IEP is even required can best be determined by examining the source of funding for the proposed program/service. Involvement in any area funded by special education requires the provision of an IEP completed prior to the initiation of the service.

4. THE PROJECTED DATES FOR INITIATION OF SERVICES AND THE ANTICIPATED DURATION OF THE SERVICES. The intent of this mandate is to provide the parents and child with a realistic prognosis of the length of time special services will be required. As such, consideration of the severity and multiplicity of the student's needs must be made and a tentative timeline established. While the IEP is reviewed and revised at least annually, the statement of duration should consider the total length of service estimated, be it throughout the entire school career, through elementary school years, or only one year, or less. It should be noted that the duration specified is not binding and can be revised according to the progress of the child.

The regulations also mandate that names of individuals who will assume responsibility for providing the needed programs and services be included on the IEP. This is required so that parents can be more cognizant of their child's program. Mandating names, however, does not make the individuals accountable for the progress of the student in their care.

While the federal guidelines do not specify how soon services must be initiated, they do indicate that the IEP should be implemented as soon as possible following the meetings held to establish or revise the IEP. Undue delay is not permissible, so in many cases it is wise to be prepared to offer the special programs and services at the time the IEP is developed.

5. APPROPRIATE OBJECTIVE CRITERIA AND EVALUATION PROCEDURES AND SCHEDULES FOR DETERMINING, ON AT LEAST AN ANNUAL BASIS, WHETHER THE SHORT-TERM INSTRUCTIONAL OBJECTIVES ARE BEING ACHIEVED. The child's special education program must be periodically evaluated in order to determine whether or not the instructional objectives are being met, whether the current placement in special education programs remains appropriate, and whether adjustments are needed to better meet the student's needs. The law mandates that this evaluation be made at least once annually, but this does not eliminate the need for periodic reports to the parents. Indeed, the parent, child, or teacher can request a new evaluation or reconsideration of the IEP at any time.

One section of the IEP form usually provides space for the educational agency to indicate when the plan will be reviewed, when or how frequently progress reports will be prepared, and/or what competencies will be evaluated. In this way, the local educational agency is held accountable for holding the review, and the parent is made aware of, and encouraged to participate in, the program planning/evaluation of the child.

Because of the requirement of gauging progress through objective evaluation, IEPs are required to contain a section correlated with the short-term objectives in which criteria for measuring each objective is listed. Such criteria may include percentage of correct responses and method of evaluation, i.e. checklists, pre-post testing, direct observation. This type of information provides both an objective vehicle for assessing progress and an intermediate step toward maintaining awareness of the current level of educational functioning.

Additionally, this federal guideline points out the need for stating annual goals and short-term instructional objectives in such a way that they can be measured easily and objectively. From this perspective, the IEP can be viewed as the accountability measure of P.L. 94-142 and will ensure that a child does not remain static over an extended period of time. Again, it should be emphasized that should the child fail to achieve the goals and objectives set out for him, the law does not hold the teacher responsible.

In addition to the provisions required by federal guidelines, several IEP components have gained widespread use. One involves identifying data, such as the student's name, address, age, grade, phone, and parents'/guardians' names. On forms used in schools or programs that accept students from other school districts, the sending school is often named. Another component typically included is a place for persons taking part in the IEP conference or annual review to sign their names, thus indicating that they are acquainted with the information the IEP contains. Some forms also provide space for the parents to indicate approval or refusal of permission for their child to participate in the proposed program.

In summary, a written individualized educational plan (IEP) must be provided for every child who is receiving or will receive special education programs and/or related services. While each local educational agency is required to develop their own IEP format, guidelines provided in P.L. 94-142 set forth components which locally developed plans must include. The IEP becomes the instrument by which the educational system assures that each handicapped youngster is receiving an individually tailored program based upon his/her unique educational needs and is being given every opportunity to participate with nonhandicapped peers to the maximum extent possible.

WHO SHOULD BE INVOLVED IN DESIGNING THE IEP?

Once the child has been assessed, and special education programming and/or services appear warranted, a meeting designed to develop the IEP in accordance with the provisions detailed in the preceding section is scheduled. In most communities, the meeting held is referred to as the placement committee meeting, while the participants are called the placement team. This same team remains involved throughout the IEP process, as they are expected to participate in the periodic or annual review conferences as well as the IEP development meetings.

Membership on the IEP team must include the child's teacher, the child's parents or guardian, the child himself whenever appropriate, and a representative of the local educational agency who is qualified to supervise the instruction or services determined appropriate for the child. Additional participants can be included at the discretion of the educational agency or the parents, although care should be taken not to include so many educators as to overwhelm the parents.

Who Should be Considered the Child's Teacher?

Selection of the teacher(s) to be involved in the IEP process is largely determined by the present placement and/or projected needs of the child. If the child is presently receiving special education, the "teacher" is usually considered the person who serves the child in the special education classroom. Representation of ancillary personnel, i.e. speech pathologist, physical education teacher, physical therapist, may be included or, indeed, serve as the primary "teacher" if the child's program includes their services.

Regular classroom teachers are often involved if the youngster has been participating in the regular program and is being considered for placement in special education, or if regular class placement is being considered for all or part of the child's school program. This is particularly important if a youngster is being phased into a vocational program, in which case a representative of the vocational department or school might wish to be involved to ensure that the student's vocational interests are met and necessary supportive services are provided. In situations where a handicapped student is totally within a vocational technical school, the responsibility for developing the IEP lies with the vocational educators; thus representation by a vocational "teacher" and administrator is necessary.

If special education programs or services are being considered for a child who has not yet entered school, or if a child has a number of teachers, the selection of the teacher(s) to serve in the IEP meetings is usually made by school administrators. This teacher is usually one who is qualified in the area of the child's suspected disability.

In most instances, the teacher(s) involved in the IEP process assumes the major responsibility for conducting the meetings, writing the actual document, and ensuring that the programs and goals are carried out. As such, a number of competencies have been identified that appear necessary for successful delivery of these responsibilities. These include:

1. the ability to identify appropriate evaluation tools, administer such instruments if permissable, and interpret the data generated;
2. competency in reporting the student's educational needs in observable, concrete ways;
3. competency in selecting and writing long- and short-term instructional goals;
4. the ability to evaluate the student's performance after intervention and to call for a review conference if revisions in the IEP appear warranted;
5. a working knowledge of the due process requirements of P.L. 94-142; and

6. the ability to communicate each of the above to parents and educational personnel.

Since many teachers may feel unprepared to meet these qualifications, these six areas provide excellent fodder for massive teacher-training efforts of the over two million "regular" teachers and 300,000 special education teachers. Such efforts are presently underway through conferences and programs offered by colleges and universities, while locally-designed in-service provided by pupil personnel administrators and/or special education supervisors address the needs on a more local level.

Involvement of the Parents

Much of the impetus behind the movement to improve the education of handicapped youngsters resulting in P.L. 94-142 came from parents, seeking not only equal and integrated educational programming for their youngsters but increased involvement and knowledge of the programs being provided. Legislation has insured this involvement by mandating that the child's parents or guardian be active participants, not mere onlookers, in determining their child's education.

It is the intent of the law that the IEP be developed in a meeting called for this expressed purpose. This ensures that input from parents be considered *before* educational decisions are made so that the observations and opinions of the parents can be incorporated into the plan. Involvement also offers parents the opportunity to monitor their child's program and to check on the progress being made. Further benefits of participation in frequent conferences include allowing the parents to get a more comprehensive understanding of their child's needs and programs, providing assistance in the development of supplementary educational experiences which will complement those being provided in school, and allowing school personnel to provide parent or family counseling services if needed.

It is the local educational agency's responsibility to notify the parents of the purpose, time, and location of the IEP meetings as well as to inform them that they may invite other people to participate. While the meetings may be conducted without the parents present, every effort must be made to secure their participation; and detailed records of these attempts must be kept. Examples of efforts made to convince the parents of the importance of their involvement include —

1. *telephone calls*: date, time, participants, and results of such efforts should be recorded, as should attempts made with no response;
2. *correspondence*: copies of letters trying to establish mutually acceptable times and locations for meetings should be kept, as well as replies to such correspondence;
3. *home visits*: date, time, and results of such visits or attempted visits should be documented.

In the event that the parents cannot or will not participate, it may be prudent to obtain a written waiver from them in which the parents document their willingness for the IEP meeting to be held without their presence. This is a legal requirement in many states and a wise precaution regardless of legal mandate.

Child Involvement

Perhaps the participant most frequently neglected in the IEP process is the youngster himself — a situation sorely in need of remediation since the primary aim of intervention and educational efforts is to assist the handicapped child (indeed *any* child) in becoming as functionally independent and responsible as possible.

Involvement of the student should be the standard rather than the exception by the time adolescence is reached, with younger children being participants if able. For who better than the individual can pinpoint what needs are present and goals are sought?

While the extent of involvement in the IEP process will be affected by the severity of the handicaps, the youngster should be an active participant in at least three areas. These include:

1. being aware of the data and assumptional bases on which educational decisions are being made;
2. providing input as to perceived strengths and weaknesses, and assisting in the selection of priorities in service; and
3. providing relevant background and personal information

that will assist other IEP team members in understanding the child more completely.

Involvement of the child can provide a number of positive results that should not be overlooked. Through participation, the youngster may realize the interest and commitment of parents and educators, thus enhancing their strength as role models. Feelings of self-worth might also be strengthened, as the child realizes that he has some input into his own destiny. Awareness of the reasons underlying approaches and the instructional goals being sought might also strengthen the child's commitment toward achievement, thereby enhancing responsibility for personal growth.

The Educational Representative

The final member required to participate on the IEP team is a representative of the local educational agency who has the authority and capability to act as spokesman for the school district in matters related to the special education programming and services the handicapped child might require. As spokesman, this member's primary responsibilities include:

1. interpreting the laws and making sure that the due process procedures are followed;
2. being aware of the programs and services available within the school district as well as those outside the system where handicapped youngsters may be served;
3. making sure that delivery of the programs/services itemized on the IEP is possible; and
4. being able to explain and implement the steps involved in expediting appropriate placement.

Since this team member is able to made decisions and placements for which the school district may be held legally and financially responsible, a special education supervisor, school psychologist, or pupil personnel director is usually selected to serve. Competencies sought in this representative include a thorough knowledge of federal and state laws, awareness of local policies and procedures, and an acquaintance with other programs which may provide services to district youth.

Other Participants

Under certain circumstances, additional participants are required at the IEP meetings, and the school system is responsible for arranging their presence. One such instance involves the provision of an interpreter for parents who have a limited mastery of the English language or who are deaf, thereby ensuring that such parents — and ultimately their youngster — are not penalized due to communication barriers.

A second situation in which an additional member is frequently involved occurs when the initial placement meeting is held. A representative from the evaluation team is expected to participate so that an explanation of the instruments and procedures used in the assessment can be provided and an interpretation of the results be made. Occasionally the teacher-member of the IEP team is competent in providing this information and therefore serves in this capacity. More commonly, however, a school psychologist or pupil personnel director is present either as an additional team member or as the administrative representative.

Whenever an IEP meeting is held, both the parents and the school district have the right to invite other individuals to participate, and it is the educational agency's responsibility to inform the parents of this right. While little can be done to control the inclusion of outside members invited by parents, additional educational personnel may be considered if their input will add breadth to the understanding of the youngster or if they will be involved in subsequent programming efforts. It should again be emphasized that the number of educators involved in the IEP process should be limited so that parents will not become overwhelmed and the committee does not become so unwieldy as to lose its effectiveness and efficiency.

IEP Responsibility

As stated earlier, the local educational agency assumes the major responsibility for ensuring compliance with the legal mandates involved in implementing individualized programs for its handicapped youngsters, state educational agencies maintain responsibility for monitoring local efforts, and the federal government exerts its influence through the provision of substantial funds for those states, and ultimately, local programs which meet the mandated guidelines. While the procedures involved differ widely, due to varying state and local policies, certain responsibilities tend to universally rest with the local pupil personnel or special education administration. These include:

1. obtaining written consent from the parents for the MFE;
2. ensuring that the unbiased, comprehensive evaluation is carried out;
3. appointing an administrative representative to serve on the IEP committees as well as selecting the teacher(s) when such responsibility is not self-evident;
4. ensuring that an interpreter is present at meetings involving deaf or non-English speaking parents;
5. contacting all participants as to the location, date, and time of the meetings, as well as the purpose of the sessions; and
6. ensuring that the IEP meeting is held, an IEP is developed, the parents' signatures are obtained, and that the programs and services identified on the IEP are implemented without undue delay.

Following the initial placement, meeting the local educational agency's responsibilities expand to include ensuring that the IEP is reviewed at least once annually and revised as needed and that a complete psychoeducational evaluation takes place at least once every three years. Clearly, the advent of P.L. 94-142 has added immeasurably to the work of special educators.

The major responsibility for providing the IEP and ensuring that the appropriate steps in the assessment, notification of participants, and due process are enforced remains with the local school district in which the child's family resides. This is so regardless of the educational program in which the handicapped child participates. Thus, responsibility for planning the program for a youngster who attends classes for the multi-handicapped in a neighboring school district (as is often the case with low-incidence programs where a number of school systems collectively offer services in one location) remains ultimately with the educational agency sending the child.

Because it is often difficult for a school district to maintain close supervision or contact with outside educational programs due to distance, sheer number of children, or unfamiliarity with programs, it is a common practice for a sending school to include a member of the receiving school's educational staff in the placement committee meeting. The wisdom of such inclusion should be immediately apparent: the home school district is legally responsible for providing any programs or services listed on the IEP and, thus, remains liable if the school where the child is sent is unable or unwilling to provide these services.

Another practice is for the local educational agency to delegate primary responsibility for the development of the IEP to the district or program actually instructing the child. This, of course, can only be done if the receiving school is willing to assume the task. Should this be the decision, a copy of the student's current IEP should still be maintained in the local school district, and every effort to participate in the IEP meetings should be made by the sending school.

Another situation which sometimes causes confusion involves the responsibility of IEP planning for the handicapped youngster who is enrolled in a vocational education program. Again, primary responsibility remains with special education and with the home district when joint vocational programs are involved.

Vocational educators should provide information to the IEP committee regarding preparation necessary for later vocational participation (skills which need to be developed in order for a child to survive in a vocational program), and a representative of the vocational program should serve on the placement committee if such placement is being considered for a youngster to ensure that the vocational placement is appropriate and that the specifications of the IEP can be provided. Development of the IEP becomes the specific responsibility of vocational education only when a handicapped student is totally served in a vocational technical school. Even then the local educational agency maintains responsibility for ensuring that all provisions are met.

CONCLUSION

While all of the ramifications of P.L. 94-142 with its stringent mandates concerning due process, evaluation, and the individualized education of handicapped students cannot yet be measured, experience within its framework is already changing, and hopefully improving, the education and treatment of the nation's handicapped population. The very procedures necessary to meet compliance with the law alter our approach to our clientele, forcing us to look beyond the disabilities exhibited by the child to a consideration of the unique social, emotional, cognitive, academic, physical, and communication strengths and weaknesses that cause him to require special services. This, in itself, may be compensation enough for the additional paperwork, conferences, and competencies thrust upon educators as a result of the law!

A number of other benefits may also be derived from the mandates. For the first time, accountability is a component of the educator's milieu, and it is possible to exert at least a degree of "quality control," since progress and programs are constantly being evaluated. The IEP process also fosters communication between the school and the community, as parents are given every opportunity to participate in the planning and implementation of their child's educational program. Psychologists and other ancillary personnel are being given a much greater opportunity to serve in a consultative role, providing in-service and counseling to both parents and teachers. There is also a much greater likelihood that there will be continuity and consistency in a child's education, as communication between programs and across age levels is required. Finally, the insistence upon an interdisciplinary approach both to the MFE and the development of the IEP allows a broad range of competencies to be tapped and encourages discussion and a genuine appraisal, from varying viewpoints, of the child's educational needs.

The advantages of the IEP, in particular, are so apparent as to cause some educational experts to forecast that someday in the not-too-distant future *all* children will be accorded the same considerations, and our schools may adopt a truly individualized approach to education.

ADDITIONAL CONSIDERATIONS

Do Regular Education Youngsters Receiving Home Instruction Require an IEP?

Yes. Tutorial services such as home instruction are provided through special education funds. As such, an IEP must be provided before home instruction can begin. This IEP should stress the suspected duration of service, areas to be covered by the tutors, and time allocations per subject.

What is the Individualized Implementation Plan (IIP)?

In recognition of the shortcomings of the IEP as a working document, many areas have developed IIPs. This extension of the IEP concentrates on writing and evaluating short-term instructional objectives and serves as a lesson plan more fully detailing the programs, specific strategies, and special materials to be used.

What Should be Done With Previous IEPs?

The local educational agency has the responsibility of maintaining copies of the IEP and its revisions so that longitudinal reviews of the student's educational program (and progress) can be gauged. Copies of past forms are typically maintained in the child's permanent records until such time they are destroyed.

Who Should Maintain Copies of Those IEPs Developed for Youngsters Attending Classes Outside the Home School District?

Current copies of the IEP should be provided to the parents, the home school district, and the district in which the child is being taught.

How Soon After the IEP is Developed Must Placement and Services Begin?

The individualized program is expected to commence as soon as possible after the IEP is developed. Unless the meetings are held during the summer or a vacation period, or unless

specific circumstances such as arranging transportation delays implementation, the child's IEP should commence immediately.

What Should be Done if a Teacher Feels a Child's IEP is Inappropriate?

Whenever a youngster enters a school system and has an IEP
which calls for services/programs that his new school feels
are inappropriate, or if a new teacher enters a district and
wishes to implement specific strategies not listed on the
child's IEP, the teacher may request that a review conference
be held for the purpose of revising the IEP. Until such a
meeting is held the existing IEP remains in effect.

What Role Does the Public School Play in the IEP Process for Children Attending Private or Parochial Schools?

Since auxiliary funds are provided to local school systems to
provide for the special education needs (including assessment) of district youngsters attending private or parochial
schools, it remains the public school's responsibility to monitor the IEPs of district students enrolled in parochial or
private schools. The local educational agency should ensure
that public school personnel chair and staff the IEP conferences, with representation from the parochial or private
schools encouraged. A copy of the IEP should be maintained
by the public school district.

What Areas Should be Addressed in the IEP?

Since the IEP is a plan for special education programs and
services, only those areas taught or funded by special education need to be included. Thus, a youngster who is receiving
special services in one area only, i.e. tutorial assistance in
math, will have an IEP limited to that area, while a child
totally served in a special education unit will have an IEP
addressing all aspects requiring attention.

What Should be Included on the IEP for a Youngster Placed in a Twenty-four-Hour Residential Facility?

The IEP is only one component in the plan for a child in a
residential program and usually addresses only those aspects
of the child's program that deal with cognitive and academic
training. A more comprehensive Individualized Habilitation

Plan (IHP) focuses on social and emotional areas as well as daily living skills. Developing the IHP is usually the responsibility of the residential facility.

Should an IEP be Developed for Pre-School Youngsters who Have Been Evaluated and Identified as Handicapped?

While school districts are responsible for locating and evaluating all handicapped residents between the ages of birth and twenty-one, the local district may not assume responsibility for educational programming for a child under age three. An IEP should be written for youngsters aged three or four only if they are to be placed in an educational program and only if this meets state laws.

REFERENCES

Education of Handicapped Children Implementation of Part B of the Education of the Handicapped Act, effective October, 1977. U.S. Office of Education Department of Health, Education, and Welfare, U.S. Govt. Print. Office,

Gibbins, Spencer. "Public law 94-142: An Impetus for Consultation." *The School Psychology Digest, 7 (3):* 18-25,

National Association of State Directors of Special Education. *Writing Individualized Assessment Reports in Special Education: A Resource Manual.* Washington, D.C. National Association of State Directors of Special Education, 1978.

State of Ohio Department of Education: *IEP* Individualized Education Program Resource Booklet.* State of Ohio: Department of Education, 1979.

"The IEP Process: How does it measure up?" *Special Education Briefing,* July/August, 1979.

INDEX